YOGA NIDRA

Traditional method to reduce stress, restore your spirit, deep relaxation and healing sleep.

Maya Soman

TABLE OF CONTENTS

INTRODUCTION

Yoga Nidra focuses on sound and mantra imagery. This kind of yoga helps to harmonize the mind and body.

The Yoga Nidra method uses the green emerald pigment. This color is famous for its calming influence. This lets you sit on the background with a picture for several minutes until the mind relaxes and calms. Usually, people use Yoga Nidra for profound relaxation.

In addition to its calming effect, Yoga Nidra is also used to relieve the back pain of pregnant women. Yoga, however, is generally a good practice for moms to boost their endurance, as their condition requires. Pregnant women with back pain can hardly foresee the time of work and childbirth during their pregnancy. Back pains are minimized with daily yoga practice. This assumption originated from the ancient Indian viewpoint on the mother's instincts and intuition. Before that, they assumed that a mother could feel the sex of the baby in the last trimester of the first child.

The basic structure of a yoga practice is breathing, posturing, and meditation. Internal stimulants, including sound and vision, however, provide a comprehensive reflection.

CHAPTER ONE:
HOW TO GET STARTED WITH YOGA NIDRA

As many wellness experts are aware, yoga Nidra is a form of yoga that can have a very beneficial effect on the health and wellbeing of a person. This form of yoga, involving a sleep-like state that causes deep relaxation, has decreased giddiness, anxiety, palpitations, headache, chest pressure, abdominal pain, and sweating. Individuals who want to use this type of yoga to improve their mental or physical health should know how to get started. Three are here:

1. Group classes can be a great way to start this kind of yoga practice, especially when someone is a beginner. You can usually go online to find the right class and search for a keyword or look through the telephone book. In some instances, people can discover types at a fitness center offering yoga classes. In other situations, people

will have to search for yoga studios to take these lessons.

2. Instructional DVDs Nearly every kind of workout, including this kind of yoga, is currently available in DVD format. Since this the case is, people who want to practice can go online and buy DVDs from a big chain store or buy them. Instructional DVDs are perfect for people who don't feel comfortable in a group setting to practice this type of yoga. Another advantage of the instructional DVDs is that you can do it whenever it suits you.

3. Personal Trainer Another alternative to begin this type of yoga is to hire a personal trainer. Such people usually have comprehensive education and experience in their profession, so that they can offer customers thorough and results-oriented assistance to promote optimal health and wellbeing. Personal coaches also work in gyms, studios, and leisure centers. Nevertheless, a lot of people work as independent entrepreneurs and can teach in your home or their private gym.

Given that most people choose to practice this kind of yoga to improve the health of their children, it is essential to note that these breathing exercises alone are not enough to achieve this goal. Alternatively, optimal health benefits from the incorporation of various activities to foster intellectual, physical, and emotional harmony. It is important to remember that this type of yoga does not involve substantial cardiovascular work, meaning that students practicing also need to include other types of exercise in their physical routine (basketball, running, cycling, taboo, kickboxing, etc.). Therefore, a balanced diet containing a significant amount of fruit and vegetables is essential to eat to achieve the nutrients required for the body and mind to function correctly. In combination, each of these activities contributes to holistic, optimal health that makes life more productive and meaningful.

All people interested in improving their health should remember that the practice of yoga Nidra is an excellent way to achieve the target. To begin, people can consider implementing one or all of the above-mentioned instructional formats. This is likely to improve people's health and allow them to lead safer happier lives.

How To Prepare For Your Yoga Nidra Class

The wellness industry is booming nowadays, as more and more people are looking for viable solutions that allow them to lead healthier lives. While a large number of health strategies can be implemented by individuals to achieve that goal, yoga practice can be especially helpful. And while there are various forms of yoga a person may engage in to improve his or her wellbeing, yoga Nidra is especially advantageous. Though broadly defined, this kind of yoga typically involves being "lied down" and then being guided by a qualified teacher through a series of breathing exercises. People who are preparing to start this form of yoga should be aware that they can do several things to make the most of it. Some of them are

1. Exercise.

This may sound like an odd piece of advice because many people opt to practice it type of yoga to find a mode of profound health relaxation. Your health optimization requires much more than conscious meditation in this type of yoga. In addition to relaxing and thus reducing or eliminating stress, people who seek optimal health must also undergo consistent cardiovascular activity. There are several forms of physical activity, including kickboxing, swimming, running, and cycling. If a couple, together with restful meditative yoga, does this type of physical activity, optimal health can be achieved.

2. Mind your sanitation. Mind your hygiene.

Good hygiene is always important, but it can be particularly important when preparing for a group yoga class. Individuals also believe that, because Nidra activities do not involve a lot of movement and sweating, there is no need to give special attention to issues such as brushing their teeth right before class and using adequate deodorant.

However, people need to do all that if they take a group yoga lesson because exercises often involve people who are close to other people. Since this is the case, please make sure before attending a class, you practice excellent hygiene.

3. Carry your bottle of water and mat.

Although people may not believe they will become thirsty because they do basic meditative yoga exercises, they will certainly. This type of mental work requires extreme concentration, often involving the use of substantial energy. Moreover, many health experts advocate drinking several ounces of water every few hours, which means that it is always essential and beneficial to keep a water bottle present . Yoga practitioners should never forget to bring a mat if they plan to practice this type of yoga in a group environment. The yoga room sometimes has all the equipment you need, but this is not always the case. Therefore, carrying a mat will prevent practitioners from experiencing the inconvenience of Nidra on a hard floor surface.

The above list is certainly not comprehensive, it does include several strategies that people can implement to prepare successfully for their yoga Nidra class. Some other strategies to consider would be to exercise consistently to avoid the irritation that may arise from less than optimal operation. The practitioners of this yoga practice should also take into account the high value of getting a partner to work with them to improve their respiration and meditation. When people incorporate some or all of these techniques in their yoga practice, they will possibly be exponentially enhanced. The result is the ability to lead a much more productive and positive life.

The Benefits of Yoga

Yoga is a theory and practices healing system. It is a mixture of breathing exercises (pranayama), physical positions (asana), deep relaxation (yoga Nidra), and meditation (Dyana).

Although Yoga has originated as a religious practice in Hinduism, it has become a purely physiological, mental, and spiritual practice in the

Western world. The majority of Western yoga practices have little or nothing to do with Hinduism. Still, they are just a way to maintain the wellness, fitness, and health of all human levels, and this is only part of a broad definition of Yoga. Through Yoga, we realize the connection between our spiritual, mental, emotional, and physical levels. This awareness gradually leads us to understand our existence's more subtle areas.

Through keeping the energy meridians (nadis) open and living energy (prana) streaming, yoga practice avoids specific diseases and diseases. Yoga is known as a mental-body treatment that decreases the effects of generalized stress on wellbeing.

Laboratory tests have shown that the yogi can actively regulate automatic or unconscious functions such as temperature, pulse, and blood pressure.

Yoga is both a preventive and curative therapy. Yoga therapy is valid according to medical scientists due to the equilibrium produced in nerve and endocrine systems that directly affect all other systems and organs of the body.

Regular practice, including acidity, allergy, Alzheimer's disease, anemia, anger, anxieties, arthritis, asthma, pain on the back, bronchitis, cancer, carpal tunnel syndrome, chronic tiredness, colitis, common cold, constipation, depression, diabetes, epilepsy, visual conditions, facial witnessing (asanas), breathing exercises (pranayama), deep relaxation (yoga Nidra) and a meditation, may help.

The physiological stage gains Increased flexibility Cure and avoid arthritis— yoga poses (asanas), operate on various joints of your body, including joints you never really use. You can experience a significant increase in flexibility in joints, ligaments, and tendons by practicing yoga poses. Yoga is paired with exercise and relaxation, and this is the perfect formula for arthritis. Slow-motion motions and gentle forces of Yoga hit the tense joints profoundly. Also, the simple stretches, together with deep breathing exercises, alleviate the stress that connects the muscles and tightens the joint further.

Healing and avoiding back pain — back pain is the most common reason for searching for medical care in the West. Yoga has been widely used by improving strength and flexibility to relieve and avoid back pain.

Relax in all of the body's essential internal organs—Research has shown that yoga poses are the only way to relax all the inner body's glands and organs, and this encourages health and wellbeing.

Total detoxification—Yoga poses (asanas) allows muscles and joints to stretch gently and ensure the best blood supplies for different parts of the body. This helps to reduce toxins from the body. This leads to advantages like aging pause, stamina, and a beautiful lifestyle.

Excellent muscle tone—Yoga practice will improve flaccid and weak muscles.

Provide equilibrium in the nervous system—yoga is a great way to meditate and to balance the nervous system.

Stress reduction-As yoga is a slow and gentle form of exercise combined with breathing exercises; stress can be alleviated.

Asthma and breathing problems Treat and prevent

Different studies have confirmed Yoga's positive effects on people with breathing problems. Doctors found that asanas, in combination with breathing exercises and meditation, are more effective in the treatment of asthma. It has also been shown that asthma attacks can usually be prevented without using drugs by yoga practice. Yoga patients have a better chance of controlling their breathing problems. With the aid of yogic respiratory exercises, an assault of extreme shortness of breath can be managed without seeking medical help.

High blood pressure (hypertension)

The primary role played by yoga postures, yoga breathing (pranayama), and deep-relief exercises (yoga Nidra) is to control or avoid higher blood pressure and to minimize the need for medications for people who experience hypotension.

Pain Management

The concentration during yoga postures, breathing, deep relaxation, and meditation can also help reduce pain. Yoga is believed to reduce pain by improving the pain center in the brain to regulate the spinal cord system and to secrete natural painkillers in the body.

Weight Reduction

Yogic activities that reduce anxiety tend to decrease stress. Regular yoga practice may help to manage weight because some asanas activate the slow gland to increase their hormonal secretions. Many asanas, such as the stand of the shoulder or the fish pose, are aimed against the thyroid gland. This glass affects our weight significantly since it influences the metabolic rate of the body. The fat metabolism is also increased so that fat is converted to muscle and energy, better muscle tone, and a higher level of vitality.

The practice of' yogic breathing' improves the absorption of oxygen in body cells, including fat cells. It leads to increased oxidation or fat cell burning.

Benefits of self-awareness

Self-awareness

Yoga practice at the psychological level increases self-awareness. The yoga practitioner learns to act rather than to react. They begin to control their feelings and learn to be aware, to live the moment, the present, and not in the past or the future.

Self-confidence

Confidence or low self-esteem is something that Yoga seeks to eliminate through practice. Someone with little regard for themselves can not do their job correctly or is quickly tired, irritable, and haggard. Anyone who practices Yoga begins to believe profoundly in themselves and their enormous potentials.

Vitality and Change of Mood

Everyone who performs Yoga over a while has a positive impact on their outward appearance and strength. Yogic postures with respiratory exercises have been shown to improve physical energy and boost mood.

Benefits for the Mental Level

Mental balancing

Common breathing (pranayama) in Yoga is the "alternative nose breathing" Electroencephalogram (EEG) research on brain electrical impulses reveals that breathing through one nose leads to increased activity on the opposite side of the brain. The regular practice of alternative nostrils contributes to better communication between the right and left brain of the brain.

Benefit for the spiritual level

Self-knowledge

The philosophy and practice of self-knowledge lead to greater self-knowledge. This expert knowledge is simply the mental part of yoga practice, which aims to cultivate and enhance the nature of the Self.

Knowing the Self, the observer, a real knowledge, tends to get lost at the hectic rhythm of our everyday lives and pursuit of desires. The discovery of the Self within us is the most valuable spiritual value in life.

Challenges of Yoga Nidra

Yoga Nidra is among the most challenging disciplines for those who want to learn it, with regular obstacles. Fortunately, the benefits outweigh any difficulties presented by the practice.

The most apparent obstacle is to fall asleep. The ideal conditions for a good Nidra session are the same as for deep, peaceful sleep. Students will probably fall into a deep state of rest at first, and this must be accepted. The desired state will occur due to time and persistence.

Another challenge is to correctly identify and differentiate the state of Nidra from other countries. The state of Yoga Nidra is so bright that it can be easier to convey an idea of the state using a negative definition and to explain what it is not.

Yoga Nidra doesn't dream lucidly. Lucid dreaming is useful as a skill, but it isn't Nidra. Meditation is also not Yoga Nidra, but meditation is undoubtedly essential to prepare the mind for such a state.

Nidra is not necessarily an alpha state in the brain and is not related to any sound or music. Recordings that claim to provide listeners with a' monk mind' within a month or a few weeks should be disregarded entirely, whether their claims are explicitly related to Yoga Nidra. Many valuable things in this life need some commitment, and deeper consciousness is no exception.

Yoga Nidra is challenging and frustrating for beginners because it is impossible to ensure that their efforts lead to the Yogic state of Nidra. In this way, Nidra's pursuit becomes a powerful spiritual practice because it cultivates a state of unbelief. Either yoga Nidra is going to happen, or it is not going to happen. No result should be attached to the student.

Except one is a Yoga teacher or an expert in meditation, Nidra may need a teacher more than any other kind of Yoga, and it can prove challenging to find a teacher who understands and knows true Yoga Nidra. A teacher helps students to instruct and use prompts such as bells or gongs to encourage a yogic Nidra state in their students. As Nidra is common in Savasana, it is easier to be guided by the sound of the voice of your teacher or by audio recording, and it is not possible to read with your eyes shut.

Yoga Nidra is an advanced practice that is worthwhile to follow, although it is worth noting that although it is different from other methods such as meditation or hatha yoga, it is not necessarily much better. Yoga Nidra, meditation, and Hatha Yoga work together well to facilitate inner transformation for practitioners, but no practice is better. These paths lead to the same reality.

Different Types of Yoga With Varying Purposes

There is more than one yoga exercise, each consisting of multiple sequences for specific physical and mental health purposes.

Kripalu Yoga: Is the best way to match posture and to blend breathing with movement. While Iyengar is a gentle form of yoga, Kundalini is another type of yoga. The former is typically used by beginners and less agile individuals, while the latter is focused on singing, meditation, visualization, breathing control, and physical positioning.

Hatha yoga: Mainly improves the flow of body movements, which makes it great for healing back pains. This is practiced in the UK. Raja Yoga and Tranta Yoga techniques are known for their ability to elevate emotions and spiritual feelings.

This emotional pleasure is understood by Yoga Nidra, considered to tap into your body and mind for its guided imaging. Yoga Nidra is integrated into its technique with the color emerald green. This is done by letting a practitioner focus for several minutes on an image with the color behind it. This color is, among other things, considered the most relaxing color.

The focus of the image will remain until the mind and body are relaxed. An audio file is also played on the background to guide meditators. Yoga Nidra regards hypnosis as a trancelike state of profound relaxation while keeping the mind alert and open. It counters the common fear of someone controlling your commercially created mind in the hypnosis idea. Like any other yoga, deep breathing and mantra are involved.

Each yoga practice has rates typical. Such rates correlate with various lifestyle aspects. First, the body is the physical, emotional, thinking mind, right-brain consciousness, left-brain awareness, personality psychology, and unconscious processes.

Anusara Yoga: Should raise awareness and provide an outstanding body, mind, and spirit with good grounding and alignment. The whole body will be toned and sensitive and, above all,-in Tune. In harmony with the universe, the source of God, your very essence and being, as you come from the heart. Express yourself through your posture and allow your heart to melt and pass through.

You will not only have a more significant, more versatile body. Consciousness will be more evident with a greater awareness that you are one.

Glen Wood: The Guru of Yoga. Glen is an expert in yoga who wants to show you how to lose the yoga pain in your arm, shoulder, and back.

Yoga For Relaxation And Relaxation Techniques For Busy People

Will you relax? Most people have a busy life and no time to relax. During their working lives, people get out of bed when they retire for the day. How can you relax when you spend the whole day following your plans, going to the office, returning home, and not having enough time to have a proper meal? Also, different types of stress may arise due to financial problems, family health issues, lack of emotional support, or pressure at work. The final result is that most of the day, you feel stressed, mentally, and physically? You desperately need rest if you feel easily irritable, energy loss, do not enjoy your job, and feel hopeless. Even if you are perfectly fine and healthy, proper relaxation can make an incredible difference in your life and reduce stress.

A person who does not do a job does not need to be relaxed. Likewise, you don't have to lie in bed when your mind is occupied elsewhere.

Is that relaxing? The activities that follow are not pure relaxation:

- Fall into a couch and watch your favorite channels. Sex, violence, and tears can add to your emotional baggage.
- A journal or magazine can make you feel better, but relaxation is not real.
- Food, drink, or party.
- You are gossiping or spreading coworkers ' gossip.
- Use of medications or any other poisonous substances.

Is it possible to relax? Yes, everyone can relax, but constructive action is needed. With continuous effort, you can master the art of relaxation. Relaxation isn't an affair once; you will continuously practice it. Make relaxation a part of your life. Do self-analysis to find any significant stress factors that can be easily solved and try to remove them. For pure leisure, the way you think is a paradigm shift. You've got to let things go. Don't think you're doing it all. Recall that you are not indispensable, the world does not rest alone on your shoulders. Here are some relaxation tips.

Yoga to relax. Yoga breathing and yoga asanas are natural stressors and improve the feeling healthy. It takes away negative feelings/emotions. Yoga helps to harmonize your mind and body and gives you more energy to work.

- Approximately 15 minutes of morning yoga practice will improve. Practice shava asana and initially rhythmic deep breathing.
- You can also practice rhythmic breathing during the day if you have at least three to five minutes of spare time. Concentrate on your breath during the day and learn about the breathing rhythm.

- In general, try to breathe deeply when you have time. Within a few days, your breathing will intensify, and you will feel the difference in emotions and the resulting mental calm.

- Yoga Nidra for complete relaxation at least once or twice a week.

Relaxation and control of the mind. Relaxation is an art that starts with a positive mental state. When you feel happy and relaxed in your account, you can contact relaxed. The mind can be conditioned for a certain period with continuous autosuggestions.

Concentration and meditation. Spend some time in solitude in a day, preferably early in the morning. Choose a room without sound or light. Try to focus your mind. Watch the thoughts as an independent observer pass through your account. After a few days of practice, try your ideas gradually. You should not allow negative thinking into your mind. It is probable, however, impractical. Develop a self-confidence attitude.

Relaxation actions. Advance your clock by 5 minutes, and most problems can be avoided. Be ready on time for all your appointments. For starters, get ready 5 minutes early before you go to the office, relax and think about the day's mission.

- Close your eyes for at least 5 to 10 deep breaths to reorder your thoughts for a short time.
- Often you quit our work for a few minutes and go to the coffee machine.
- Take the stairs and go up to the next floor.
- Sleeping on a good night is essential for better relaxation and helps to avoid sleep deprivation.
- Perhaps your daily routine changes. Sometimes go for a long walk in a nearby park, for example. Spend some time in nature's lap.
- Develop a hobby like yoga, meditation, running, swimming, or gardening.

Relaxation feelings.

- You do not need the approval of others for all your acts, so be confident and don't worry what others think about you.

- You can relax while doing your job, if you like your work and work fully.

- Don't think about your past or your future.

- Every day, spend some time with your family. Your family can offer you the emotional support you need.

- You can also find pleasant memories in yourself to help you relax.

- Yes, it is essential to have a happy married life and a harmonious atmosphere at home for peace of mind.

Monitor your breathing and heart rate by rhythmic breathing so that in all situations, you can remain calm and composed. Relaxation involves defining and prioritizing the main work and completely disregarding irrelevant issues. Practicing these relaxation techniques will allow you to concentrate on relevant questions, enhance productivity at work, and lead a healthy life.

Yoga Nidra For Stress Reduction & Deep Relaxation

Stop a moment and wonder: does stress have a real impact on my health? If it's "No," think again. Medical researchers estimate that up to 90% of disease and disease are related to stress. Everything so slight as cold to the more paralyzing heart disease and cancer can be complicit in pressure. Many people claim that, whether you work too much or not, you still build up physical, mental, and emotional stress. While yoga may undoubtedly help, stress and anxiety go deep and may need more focus.

You can call Yoga Nidra here. Over thirty years ago, Swami Satyananda Saraswati, founder of the renowned Bihar School of Yoga in East India, adapted old techniques of tantric meditation to the practice he called "yoga Nidra," which he describes as "psychic sleep." The Swami calls the prolonged suspension from Yoga Nidra's vigilance and sleeps a "hypnogogic state," which attests to the innumerable and extensive benefits of this place. Here can awaken our highest levels of imagination and healing energies.

In this condition, one can finally change thinking— and even personality— for the better. Yogis throughout the years have learned this through the technique of purification of sanskaras or the profound experiences and ingrained habits that cause our normal negative responses. Even if profound transformation is not your goal, you will be glad to know that you come from Yoga Nidra and feel rested and ready to enter the world (the equivalent of about 3 hours of deep sleep is said to be a twenty-30 minute session of Yoga Nidra!).

This is good news, sponsored by Daniel N. Guerra, Psy. D, Clinical Stress Management Services Director in New York City. "We've lost a much-needed connection to our minds and bodies in this fast-paced world in which we live," he explains, "Yoga Nidra helps restore the connection and is beneficial on many levels. It gives muscle relaxation, better understanding, control over our emotions, and improves psychological health." In the first stage of the session, muscles are slowly relaxed by quickly shifting consciousness during various parts of the body. The Swami drew this from the old tantric Nyasa practice (meaning' to place' or' to think about that'). The following are further tantric meditations: awaking the sensations of opposites; consciousness of the entire body, brain, and internal organs; and experiencing the bond between the world and body. Then you can be asked to focus and uniquely count your breath. In the final step, representations from nature and abstract symbols are easily visualized.

The Swami, a keen scientist, unravels the logic behind every point. From a neurophysiological viewpoint, he describes that all part of the body has a corresponding brain control center called the motor homunculus. The consciousness movement across several parts of the body not only relaxes them but also clears the nerve pathways to their parallel areas in this part of the brain. One consequence is a less fractured consciousness.

First, opposite meditation activates the centers of the brain that maintain equilibrium between the inner and outer worlds. This helps balance our fundamental drives. Finally, when the conscious mind is asked to visualize these symbols quickly, it has no time to respond. You remain detached, and the ego temporarily becomes inactive. This process helps overcome deleted conflicts, wishes, recollections, and sanskaras.

At the beginning and end of each session, you will be asked to repeat or resolve a Sankalpa. It should be a short, positive-language statement in the current tense. Pick something you want to grow that will have a positive effect on your life.

Yoga Nidra for Sleep Disorders

Most people in our contemporary society have trouble consistently sleeping well. It is estimated that 50% of adults are battling insomnia in the United States. The manifestations of insomnia vary from sleeping problems too often waking at night to getting up too early. Many factors can lead to insomnia. An individual may have sleeplessness due to a medical condition like sleep apnea, restless leg syndrome, or periodic limb movement. Insomnia can also be caused by stress, anxiety, an overactive nervous system, and depression.

Yoga Nidra is an old technique of Yoga that can help address many of the underlying causes of insomnia. Nidra exercises help balance an overactive nervous system and emotional anxiety. Nevertheless, Yoga Nidra practice does not fix all physical or medical insomnia causes. If you think that your insomnia may be due to a medical condition, you should visit your doctor to see the exact cause and treatment of your sleep problem. For example, you may need to have a breathing system at night if you have sleep apnea.

Yoga Nidra methods aid healing by fostering a deep sense of calm and well-being that helps to re-establish spiritual, mental, and physical wellness. Yoga Nidra techniques help the two hemispheres of the brain as well as the parasympathetic nervous systems to balance. During a Yoga Nidra Session, unresolved emotional issues are also dealt with by creating images and sensations that cause pain, frustration, and anxiety while enabling the thoughts, pictures, and experiences to go.

A too held nervous system and the presence of unresolved emotional problems contribute significantly to insomnia. Yoga Nidra techniques are used through several exercises to address these problems and rebalance both the brain and the nervous system. A typical session usually begins with mild yoga asanas and the setting of a Sankalpa. This old set of techniques leads the practitioner through a rotation of consciousness of all the fields of the body, gradual relaxation, breath consciousness, emotional integration, meditation, or Dharana, with an overview of the original Sankalpa. A big Nidra session will take a Yoga practitioner to a profound state of incorporation, relaxation, and relationship with the Divine.

CHAPTER TWO:
YOGA NIDRA AND THE INSOMNIA EPIDEMIC

Have you ever wondered how insomnia has become such a significant problem? Auto accidents may get the headlines for lack of sleep. Still, the Center for Disease Control reports that the number of Americans suffering from sleep deprivation is rising to be an epidemic in public health. People who can not sleep, are more susceptible to accidents, more sensitive to health problems, more vulnerable to interactive challenges, and more susceptible to anxiety and depression. Although insomnia is more frequent in women than in men, it affects genders and people of all ages.

Sleep deficiency disturbs metabolism, weakens the immune system, and contributes to the intolerance of insulin, obesity, and arterial irritation. The good news is that the regular practice of Yoga helps to counter many of these problems, particularly when asana and breathing with Yoga Nidra are combined.

Nidra in Sanskrit means sleep, but in recent years it has taken on its reputation as a method of relaxation. This is not an accurate description because Yoga Nidra describes an awake state of consciousness, but its most profoundly relaxed state. The thought brain is in charge during an average day - it responds to all five senses and pays no attention to the subconscious. However, when the mind and the body relax, the subconscious surfaces can take over the natural and creative parts of the brain.

That is what happens in the practice of Nidra. The mind loses its connections with the physical body and ego when brain waves enter an altered state. Self-defeating doubts and concerns will disappear in this extended state, and healing will take place. The mind is calm, and sleep quality enhances. Once we wake, the feelings of tiredness and distress are lost by meditation as physical, mental, and emotional stress is released.

At least one study has found that the rest can be up to four hours of regular sleep within one hour of Yogic sleep. Nidra also reduces in the following ways sleep deprivation.

• Improves sleep quality.

• Help reduce stress and control illnesses associated with stress.

• Support reduces medication requirements.

• It is recommended for psychosomatic disease prevention.

•It reduces sleep disorder symptoms and restless leg syndrome.

While Yoga Nidra rejuvenates and calms the physical body, the effects are even more profound. It produces a state of consciousness that helps to release negative patterns of thought and habits from the past, clearing the mind to sleep in the right night and to have positive feelings for life.

Using Yoga Nidra To Combat Night Terrors

Western physicians have now been investigating a Yoga Nidra practice, which means' Yogic sleep,' an all-natural, holistic way to achieve an uninterrupted, relaxed, and healthy nightly sleep. It can even be a successful treatment for night terrors and severe other sleep disturbances.

Western physicians now study a practice called Yoga Nidra, which means' yogic sleep.' This tantric approach is a usual, holistic way to get a restless sleep every night. It can even be a successful therapy for night terrors and other severe sleep disturbances.

The name night terrors are a severe threat to sleep. The relatives of night attackers are often terrified and confused. During an episode, a person sleeps for one moment, then stands abruptly, screaming or shuddering in the middle of the bed.

During the night, a person may look wild, sweating, and breathing around the room. You may cry uncomfortably, scream in terror, or run around the room. Nevertheless, they remain sleeping during the episode, unaware of the chaos that they create.

Only a small number of children and even smaller adults suffer night terrors. While children generally overcome night terror, the problem often persists into adulthood.

This tantric form, to promote restful sleep, is translated from Sanskrit into yogic sleep. It is a highly advanced method to facilitate deep, full relaxation.

The calming technique involves mental imagery of 20 to 45 minutes led by an experienced coach. Finally, the subject enters a profound meditative state. This state will release negative emotions and thought patterns, calm the nervous system, and lead to sleep, the yoga community believes.

The practice can also work for the following conditions, including

- Troubled sleep
- Insomnia
- Chronic pain

- Chemical dependency
- Post-traumatic stress disorder
- Why This program will function with sleep disorders

In a strictly sequential order controlled exercises center a person's mind on their entire body. The recommended order follows a systematic road to optimal relaxation. Those who use the yogic system find that evening practice makes it easier to reach this relaxed state.

Some tantric masters reach a changed sleep state known as waking sleep. A deep trance is required to get to the waking state of rest. In the stupor, the master of yoga sleeps peacefully while still being fully aware of the immediate environment. Legend has it that an hour's sleep is the same as several hours ' healthy sleep.

There are no obvious safety risks as a result of the use of this Yogic Sleep Method. The treatments are drug-free, which reduces the risk of bad experiences or dependencies. Also, children can use this device safely.

For those who have night terrors or other sleep disturbances, this device could be used for a short trial for several months. Local yoga studios could have experienced instructors using the guided imaging techniques of the system. If there are no nearby courses, some teachers have registered online workshops. You can use CDs or digital recordings every night at the bedside by a personal guide.

For everyone, from a pre-school person to a centennial, the Yoga Nidra practice is secure and safe. Who knows? Who knows? It could only work! It is certainly worth trying to have enough restful sleep every night.

Yoga Nidra, a Simple Practice for the Advanced Being

For different reasons, we all come to yoga. However, traditionally you don't go to yoga to lose a few pounds. According to the Eight Limbs of Yoga, all guidelines on personal and universal conduct are followed before you enter Asanas-the exercises, most of us associate with yoga today. After Asanas, the old text says one should practice

Pranayamas or energy management by control of the breath. Then we get to Pratyahara, where we can quickly observe interactions beyond the physical and psychosomatic diseases at their heart. For instance:

Do you suffer from this?

- Stress
- Depression
- Anxiety
- Out of night
- Bowel irritable
- Ulcer Peptic
- Migraines

Yoga Nidra, a technique that is part of Pratyahara, could help you.

As modern medicine continues to advance the cure of previously untreatable bacterial and viral infections, our rapidly evolving culture has just generated unprecedented psychosomatic diseases. These conditions are often more pronounced among those who live in congested urban centers, causing disasters on quality of life. Contemporary medicine prescribes drugs and procedures to relieve symptoms, but new methodologies often hold the root cause.

Yoga Nidra is a traditional approach to therapy that is central to the problem. Swami Satyananda Saraswati of Bihar University originally developed the Yoga Nidra, when the mind is unusually receptive and in a state between waking and sleep. It is suitable for all, regardless of fitness levels. Previous yoga experience is not mandatory.

But beware: there is a twisted understanding that decreases the power of the yoga Nidra experience, and meaningful but uneducated new agents think that yoga Nidra is just the asleep assistant. In the first, the development of a Sankalpa or a determination, and then a rotation of consciousness designed to stimulate specific areas on the cortical homunculus in the brain, two hallmarks indicate that you are getting the traditional, therapeutic Yoga Nidra taught through Satyananda and Bihar tradition. Eventually, explicit instruction should be issued not to fall asleep and remain alert without concentration.

As you are a fervent Yoga Nidra practitioner and have the highest respect for the heritage of Bihar University, I am pleased to present workshops on Yoga Nidra throughout Asia. We explore how the daily stresses in the body and mind accumulate in an intimate, fun, and therapeutic environment. Although Yoga Nidra is not a cure for a specific illness, its deep relaxation and peace of mind open the way to vibrant wellness.

Ways to Reduce Stress in Ten Minutes

Stress management is so standard that for most people, it has become a daily practice. Stress (also known as anxiety) is defined as a reaction to an incentive that disturbs our physical or mental strength. This is a broad definition that can include a lot. Stress is humorous because it's subjective. For one person, what can be stressful is a breeze for another. The bad thing is that you don't always know when it comes; otherwise, you can prepare it. The good thing is it can be handled.

Stress is a reaction, as mentioned. It's not a snapshot. It's not automatic, in other words. You can, therefore, choose how you respond to the stimulus. As it stands, the average person initially reacts negatively to stress and then changes course. This leads to animosity and acts or comments that are regrettable later but need not be so. You can prevent embarrassments, mistakes, and accidents associated with antagonistic anxiety responses by learning how to handle them effectively.

1. Focus-At the beginning of a stressful situation, the best thing you can do is focus. Don't talk but concentrate. Speak as little as possible and try to control your tone if you need to answer. Speak louder and louder. Therefore, whether you address a person or a group of people at the time, the incident will not become an insult. While conflict can catalyze change, it is a disaster recipe if you are in a warm environment. Excuse yourself if the time is right to be alone.

The goal here is to organize the mind and the emotions that move through it. You can do this through meditation. Meditation can be anywhere. it is not necessary to sit in the middle of the floor, crossing your legs, and your eyes close, but you have to get to a quiet place to stay for yourself. Try to find an object to concentrate on, and then count until you feel calm. If you want to close your eyes, do that. Visualize the number in your mind as you count — for example, count 1, 2, 3-1 in this way. When you think about the name, could you give it a mental picture? This will make you concentrate further and drive out other distractions from your awareness.

2. Journal-If your thing is not meditation, try to log your feelings. You only need a piece of paper and a utensil to compose. You can type your sentiments on your screen or the notepad on your telephone if you prefer. It is good news because it allows you to get things out of your chest and mind without striking at the people around you. There are no journaling rules. You can say what you want, who you want, how you want. And as this document is

only for you, you do not need to worry about offending or politically correcting anyone. Just write until you get everything out.

It would help if you didn't remember only how you felt, but what made you feel like that. Is it someone who said or sent you into a state of rage? Or was it something you haven't done? Do not apologize for how you feel, but take your part in ownership. When you're done, you can throw away or erase the text; it's your choice. When you decide to keep it, take the time to return to your entries at a later date. You're going to learn some stuff about yourself. You can also find patterns of those with whom you frequently connect. This can help you manage similar stressors more efficiently in the future.

3. Listen to Music- "Lose yourself in the right music is an immediate and effortless way of reworking your situation." It can be used to stimulate, motivate, or relax. Music therapy has more attention and affects pain management, stress, behavioral disorders, and even autism, but you don't require a formal study to prove its

efficacy. Know your circumstances. If somebody were to play a particular song from a few years ago, you might say correctly what you were doing, with whom you were and perhaps even what you were wearing. Music is mighty. It calls on your emotions. It's talking to us.

Once, the aim is to coordinate your thoughts in the face of a stressful situation. If possible, you want to turn it into something positive or nothing at all. Listen to something mellow. See something mellow. Classical music has demonstrated its efficiency. If you don't like Bach or Mozart or if you are too soothing, try some smooth jazz, ideally instrumental. Words or lyrics of songs can turn into a diversion. Consider gospel music if you want to hear words of encouragement. This not only has the power to calm, but the words inspire you. It gives you energy and compassion and helps you to take things into account.

4. Exercise-physical activity is an excellent way to depression as endorphins are released. Endorphins are "morphine's like a body drug." In other words, the body has an internal coping

mechanism to make you experience euphoria and push past pain. Serotonin, another mood raising substance created by your body, is also released. You can use this information to reduce stress. Nonetheless, you have to exercise at a consistent rate to benefit from these natural defenses (by exercise).

Try aerobics, long-distance running, swimming, or cycling for the best results. These activities raise your heart rate and require you to concentrate. This way, you can take your mind fully off the issue or allow you to think more clearly. After exercise, you're more ready to find ways to respond positively to the stress or problem. Boxing and basketball are other activities to try. Although neither involves constant motion, they require high heat levels and safe methods of pout attack.

5. Eat-Eating can and reduces stress while emotional eating is frowned on. This isn't an excuse for Ben and Jerry to spend a half-gallon (there are parameters for this procedure), but some foods are a healthy treat. You can see that the body has neurotransmitters called serotonin in

addition to endorphins. You will find serotonin in your intestine and central nervous system. It controls bowel movement, sleep, muscle movement, appetite, and mood.

Eat a complex carbohydrate to produce serotonin naturally in your brain. This will create a calm feeling over you. Stay away from simple carbohydrates (sugar stuff). Stay away. Even if you are rushed, the surge of energy is combated with exhaustion and fatigue. Make sure that whatever you eat is low in fat and try to do it empty-mindedly. The chocolate is the right choice. Some are a Turkish sandwich on whole wheat or your favorite spicy sauce. Protein increases alertness, so mixing carbs and protein not only can calm you down, but it can also help you develop a Stress Management Plan.

Natural Ways to Reduce Stress and Anxiety
The effects of stress can be huge, with both short- and long-term consequences. Stress may influence eating habits and sleep cycles and lead to low metabolism and inactivity. Pressure can also increase poor habits, such as smoking and

drinking, leading to significant health problems, such as cancer and heart disease. Stress hormones like cortisol deplete the body of vitamins B, C, A, and magnesium that becomes used to tension the muscles and increase blood pressure in stress reactions. B vitamins that help maintain our nerves and brain cells are mostly needed during times of anxiety. If calories consumed during times of stress do not come from nutritious foods, the vitamins are diminished even faster. Even a slight deficiency of vitamin B over a few days after consumption of empty calories such as chips and soda can disrupt the nervous system and stress. In times of stress, try consuming bananas, fish, baked potatoes, avocados, chicken, and dark green leafy veggies, all of which constitute great vitamin B sources.

B Complex Vitamins-B vitamins have been shown to have a direct impact on brain neurotransmitters such as serotonin, norepinephrine, and dopamine. Evidence suggests, in the balance and metabolism of neurotoxic chemicals linked to anxiety and depression conditions, that B-vitamins are essential. B vitamins maintain the surreal glands and become consumed during the "fight or flight" reaction when food is converted into body energy. We like Hi-Power B Complex Capsules Natural Factors.

Glutamine- The most abundant muscle cell amino acid protects muscle by reducing cortisol levels.

Inositol- Has have been shown to help cortisol reduction in patients with mental disorders like anxiety and OCD.

L Theanine- A common amino acid derivative found in tea, can cross the blood-brain barrier. Theanine has psychoactive properties, and mental and physical stress reduction has been shown. L-theanine can help the body to respond to infections by enhancing the capacity of gamma delta T cells to combat disease.

Magnesium- is present in your cells and bones and is particularly crucial for protecting the arteries against stress. Food sources include dark green vegetables, whole grains of brown rice and whole bread of wheat, garlic, lemon, avocado, chamomile, cantaloupe, black beans, and seeds of pumpkin seed and chocolate in particular. If you are overly stressed, even if you consume these foods regularly, you might become magnesium deficient.

If the body's hormonal response is stressed for any reason, it causes magnesium from the cells to flow into the blood. The greater the pain, the higher the loss of magnesium. The lower your magnesium level, the more reactive you will be to stress, which causes more significant cell magnesium loss (the higher your hormone adrenalin and cortisol levels in stressful situations).

Soaking an Epsom salt bath can help. Magnesium acid salts, including magnesium chloride, citrate, gluconate, and glycinate, are the safest dietary supplements. We like Calcium & Magnesium Citrate Plus D Natural Factors.

Omega 3 fatty acids- The central nervous system was thought to have a calming effect. We prefer Nordic DHA in the taste of strawberries.

Phosphatidylserine (PS)- Is a cortisol blocker that drives nutrients into your cells and removes toxins. It can help to avoid short-term loss of memory, age-related dementia, and Alzheimer's disease.

Vitamin C– Long tension reduces adrenal vitamin C and increases blood concentrations. We suggest 1-2 grams with food three times per day. In January 2007, Psychology Today reported that the impact of Vitamin C on the human body is subtle. Vitamin C is water-soluble, so the risk of taking large doses is low.

In reducing the level of cortisol, the following can help early bedtime

- Try to sleep around 10 pm, insufficient sleep is a stressor causing too much cortisol. Melatonin is a natural sleep help that can help you to re-establish your sleep cycle.
- Hypnosis can also be beneficial in sleep induction and a feeling of comfort.
- Eat frequently- Your cortisol levels increase after five hours without food, and you feel

"famine" when you eat, and you go into storage mode. An excellent way to prevent excessive fat storage is throughout the day to eat small meals.

- Eat protein-containing breakfast— protein helps to restore glycogen reserves required to fuel your brain. After sleep, your mind is particularly exhausted.

- Remove sugar and processed foods-eat plenty of fruits and vegetables to ensure vitamins increase your stress resistance. Particularly noteworthy are vitamins C, B1, and B2, see below.

- Eliminate caffeine-caffeine directly stimulates adrenaline and cortisol stress hormones. Caffeine is a diuretic; it depletes your water body and vitamins and leads to bone loss. Caffeine can also affect sleep quality.

- Drink water-dehydration induces a stress response that increases the level of cortisol. Drink water before going to bed and waking up.

- Minimize extensive physical activity-your body can lose testosterone levels after one hour of exercise, and cortisol starts to rise. Keep training for less than an hour and not practice for more than two days in a row.
- Practice some relaxing activities like massage, sex, and laughter.

Here are some additional tips to improve your sense of wellbeing:

- Fresh air- Break your mind and body from sitting and looking at your computer. Try to get out during the day at least once.
- Exercise—behaviors with low impacts such as walking or rollerblading are sufficient to produce endorphins without stressing the body.
- Reduce your morning commute-studies in people with long morning commutes show higher levels of cortisol. The use of public transport instead of driving will reduce traffic jams tension. Some activities that can

make your travel more enjoyable include carpooling, music, and the option of a slightly longer but less crowded route.

- Hypnosis and self-hypnosis-hypnosis of stress can be very beneficial for relaxation and can also be used as a natural way to sleep.

- Deep breathing- Faint or irregular pattern of breath caused by stress can interfere with the balance of oxygen and carbon dioxide. During tension, excess carbon dioxide can be expelled by breathing out five long seconds and then refilling your lungs naturally (do not breathe consciously). Do this in a row with a closed mouth for five respirations, and you should feel calm. Regular deep respiration can prevent illness, as the duller air you exhale, the fresher air you can inhale, which goes deeper into your lungs and doesn't provide a moist, damp environment for multiplying all the dull crawls.

- You are who you encircle yourself with Love and Positivity. Choose quality instead of quantity when it comes to friendships and surround yourself with people who inspire you. For some, the effects of drama and gossip can be a significant source of stress.

- Retract your thinking patterns— it goes beyond just trying to see the bright side of things. The mind will affect the immune system directly. "The brain has the capacity for peripheral modulation.

How Does Smoking Cigarettes Reduce Stress?

It is said that cigarettes help reduce stress and help people relax, and when smokers ask why they cannot stop smoking, they regularly produce a fact. "I can't stop being stressed too much." It is a typical sentence a smoker uttered every day by many. And if a smoker is in a complicated, confusing, critical, and anxious situation, he more than probably needs a cigarette to relax his nerves.

And smokers also receive several other benefits from smoking, including increased concentration, an additional' energy' mental strength to cure boredom and relaxation.

These aspects can be categories into two main advantageous smoking areas. First, it's soothing and relaxing to smoke, and second, it helps smokers concentrate and think clearly.

On the calming and relaxing side, cigarettes remove stress (relaxation) from their lives and relieve tension and stress. Smoking helps to relax smokers and decreases anxiety and stress. When you imagine what's up to you or talk about relaxing? Typically, it's a slumping impact of the shoulders. Slip into your armchair and let the feeling go-relax.

Smoking is uplifting on the strength and boosts side, contributes to concentration, maintains smokers on their heads, and gives them a mental toughness. The other downside of smoking is that they lift smokers to a certain level-their sense are awakened. When you visualize or think about concentrating and uplifting yourself, what does it mean? It's usually a head up on our feet, open eyes, chest out, back of shoulders, and an alert of mind and impact. It lets you be comfortable; let's do it, and makes feel.

So cigarettes can have two consequences — cigarettes can sometimes make you feel more relaxed and calmer— a general sense of calmness or peacefulness. AND a cigarette can make you feel more comfortable, competent, better equipped to handle stressful situations, and can give you an enthusiastic and inspired feeling.

But how can both these things be achieved by this same commodity or substance?

Smokers have been advised that cigarettes not only help to reduce tension but also keep you up to date- two wholly different results. Relaxation is a feeling of suppression and concentration of a sense of elevation.

How can the same material or product make the body feel comfortable and relax and increase inner peace?

In reality, cigarettes can't or can't help smokers to do both, or they can't.

It was also said that cigarettes could cure boredom, allow you to enjoy your coffee, tea, and food, and have sex more.

But again, how can cigarettes do all that? Yes, nicotine is stimulating (when dopamine, a natural pleasure drug for the body, is emitted into the brain), but how does hell make you feel up and down?

Essentially, you said cigarettes could do almost anything you want, depending on the circumstances around you while you smoke. If you need mental energy or power, then you should also have a smoke, and you would like to relax and forget about your problems. How can you sound like the same smoke, depending on your choice?

The fact is that all the other substances in the cigarette stress your brain and body-despite nicotine, which releases dopamine into the brain-make you feel more tense, more anxious, stressed, and more on the edge of the mind. It's the cold hard truth no matter how much you argue against that!

See the undeniable stressful effects of smoking on yourself and your body.

1. When you enter your body, carbon monoxide and nicotine reduce your brain's amount and supply of oxygen. Without this oxygen (the brain fuel), your mind has difficulty working correctly, thinking clearly, and focusing.

It is a fact that the level of nicotine and carbon monoxide in a smoker's body decreases, and it is also a fact that the body requires oxygen to concentrate.

Oxygen is the foundation of all body activity-all efforts made by the body (from thinking to running) are harder with less oxygen. Cigarette carbon monoxide and nicotine prevent the brain, and another organ from reaching oxygen-it cannot help to relax or concentrate. It's impossible! It's impossible!

The nicotine may make you pick me up, but it and the cigarettes only can't do everything millions of smokers have to believe and tell you.

2. This shrinks your veins and arteries in size, which means that your heart must work harder, but through a smaller space, to pump the same amount of blood across your body. Therefore, tar and other cigarette chemicals are accumulated in your veins, which further reduces blood flow.

The result is that 35,000 times more your beats per day than a non-smoker and 10-20 points higher your blood pressure than it should be under this added workload.

3. The effect of nicotine on your blood insulin places your body under constant stress. If you smoke every forty-five minutes, nicotine in the body inhibits the release of insulin (this is the suppressive influence of appetite).

Once this nicotine is burned out, the insulin is rereleased, and you have another cigarette 40 five minutes an hour or two later.

This stop-start process places enormous strain on your body-if a non-smoker's body doesn't eat insulin flow in a while; he will reduce it only when he needs it. But smokers start their body 20 times more or more a day than a non-smoker. This is an additional stressful workload.

4. Many thousands of chemical substances, poisons, toxins, and carcinogens force the body into a state of shock by cigarettes.

If you inhale cigarette smoke, your body must adapt to the presence of harmful chemicals. Everyone deposited in the veins, lungs, heart, arteries, and other organs of your body are best cleared of foreign materials when you stop smoking for a few hours (e.g., at night).

Cough of the smoker also experiences this process during the day, when your body has had eight hours or so to begin the cleansing process, and you have a significant number of mucus.

Both these cleaning practices put your body through a problematic cleansing procedure every day you stop smoking every day of your life. A non-smoker is cleansed just as extensively as a smoker if he has a virus or infection or smokes a cigarette.

The reality is that cigarettes and nicotine can only be used for' active' stress relief. And that's the key–you think.

All comes back to what you think. You think they do because you tell yourself cigarettes relax you. You think they do (although you put a great deal of strain on your system-you have an extra 35.000 times daily heartbeat because of the reduction in the venous size which makes your blood pressure higher).

Thus, while cigarettes and nicotine have a harmful and debilitating effect on your body that you have always known, you believe they strengthen and empower you to deal with life. It's a smart trick the tobacco companies pulled on you!

They have shown on films, TVs, and advertisements that cigarettes help you to concentrate, revive stress, beat problems, enjoy sex more and make men male and women sexier.

You must give them credit because it worked, and it still works! But once you take a step back, you can see that advertising and your beliefs have led you to believe that you need cigarettes and nicotine and that they have many advantages if that's all in your head!

But can't it be the placebo effect that makes you concentrate and relax? (believes something will happen, makes it happen) The truth is no but to some degree.

Yeah, you can feel very comfortable when you smoke, that's how you respire when you smoke. Have you noticed a difference in your smoking breathing? Take a moment and put your fingers on your lips to suggest that you are smoking, or better yet-light a cigarette!

Have you found anything other than your standard breathing patterns? You should have noted the two trends below.

First of all, your respiration was much stronger when you smoke. Try it again, inhale it, as if you had a cigarette smoking. This deeper respiration sucks much more air than normal breathing because you suck air from the bottom of the belly (the diaphragm of your body). This additional air also provides more oxygen-your brain and body fuel **up to 20% more oxygen** than when you usually breathe.

The second thing you ought to have noticed is how you exhale. Your air was also much stronger and more profound when you smoke. Try it again, breathe out profoundly without smoke, do it a lot.

How do you feel? How do you think? You don't feel relaxed and calm! **Exhalation feels good, mainly when done actively**. Did you notice that you exhale and breathe out forcefully when you laugh and sigh? Breathing out affects the body in a calming and positive way. So even if the smoke puts a strain on your body, you feel good when you breathe out.

So, you do deep breathing exercises when you smoke. The deep breaths give more oxygen to your body and organ, helping you to relax and release stress to some extent.

Smoking itself also doesn't reduce stress or allow you to focus on any way that's the way you breathe. Have you ever wondered why people urge you to breathe deeply if you experience symptoms of hunger or abstention? This is because the deep respiration imitates the way you breathe when you smoke.

You put your body under stress every time you have a cigarette. Then your body tries to clean up the chemicals, which makes you feel uncomfortable again and stresses. And you go around and around in circles every day, no wonder you're so stressed out!

Then you get pangs and craves when you know that your body has intense low blood sugar, (no nicotine to block insulin that activates the sugar shops) because your body needs sugar-it gets stressed. Then you have a cigarette to alleviate this stress. Then the process begins again after forty-five minutes or so! You wander around in a vast circle that is damaging and meaningless.

Smoking is said to reduce stress when, in fact, when nicotine and the chemicals enter your body, you put it under an enormous strain. Then it becomes stressful when the nicotine leaves the body because there is no nicotine to release sugar into the blood.

Tobacco induces depression and then relieves it when you smoke (artificially by playing with blood sugar levels). Smoking is like tobacco with a hammer over your mouth because when you quit, it feels perfect!

One of the main reasons why people say they can't stop smoking is because they feel that they'd give up a highly effective stress management technique. But once you stop smoking for a short time, you're calmer than if you were a smoker, even under stress.

Another smoking myth is that it' heals boring,' so meaningless that it does not deserve much attention. Yeah, some people think that it prevents boredom, but it slams your head against a wall and buckles you with a fork. This does not mean that it is either good for you, reliable, efficient, or the right way of dealing with the situation.

Again, all you do is tell yourself, if you rely on cigarettes to cure boredom-' I am not good enough to handle this situation by myself. My cigarettes take care of it. "If you smoke due to boredom, you have to take special care to change your habits to keep you entertained.

Smoking as a mechanism for stress relief is right and right. Most smokers know this, but they still lie to themselves, for they don't admit that they can't stop smoking.

Ways to Manage and Reduce Stress
There have always been just 24 hours a day and 365 days a year, but more people seem to be trying to pack up every hour, minute, and day than ever before. The more it is achieved, the higher the level of future expectations. If demands of a person's

time are that, the desire to do so increases and tension, anxiety, or depression sometimes results — none of the three things anybody wants. Stress and anxiety are the easiest to handle, however. Depression is an extremely severe medical condition. Depression is a common problem in mental health and differs significantly from mere disappointment or sadness. Depression is related to changes in the concentration of certain brain chemicals. These changes can make it very difficult for depression to break out without treatment. Stress is usually not as acute as depression, and importance is discussed here. It is clear.

Stress is the modern age's most common food. The cause of peptic ulcers, heart disease, depression, autoimmune disease, asthma, diabetes, and even cancer was found to be included. Stress is experienced when the demands on available resources are imbalanced with our ability to meet these requirements. Weight can be defined as a state of "mental or emotional strain or suspense" in its most straightforward words. Stress is not a diagnosis but is a process. Stress is often defined as a non-specific stimulus-response and is regarded by many as tension and irritation. In our lives, we all need a certain amount of weight. A small amount is healthy and helpful. In a study by over ninety companies, Watson Wyatt, a consultant company and trusted business partner of the world's leading employee and financial organizations, stated that stress is the leading cause of employees leaving work.

Stress is so significant because, in particular, situations, it brings with it feelings of loss of control or lack of choice. This lack of control makes people feel trapped, worried, and often helpless to influence change. Stress and its consequences are essential factors in mental illness, particularly anxiety and depression. Feelings of stress or anxiety warn the nervous system to respond to "battle or flight," marked by low respiration, elevated blood pressure and heart rate, and increased muscle strain.

Now that the exact stress and the more dangerous the more severe cases are established; the question becomes what can be done about them? First of all, in your life, create "flexible control." Know that all the details of your life can not be controlled. Life is unpredictable, and things sometimes happen that are not controlled by you. The growth of self-acceptance will benefit in many ways. One of the main reasons is that this avoids the negative impact of low self-esteem and self-worth.

Here are a few successful breakthroughs to rising stress levels in your life so that you can use the positive and moderate stress levels in your life to warn you about issues that you need to be vigilant about. When your body gives you these alerts, it's essential to listen.

1. Short explosions of meditation, daydreaming, sitting with a cup of tea, or even just staring at the window, will calm down and lower stress.

2. Get up every morning, fifteen minutes earlier. It gives you more time to eat something, find anything you've missed, or have a cup of coffee before leaving the door.

3. Write it down. Write it down. Write down goals, orders, tasks, project dates, and library books. Keep a "Do" list as well as a "To Do" list.

4. Allow a desire something unusual and completely unexpected.

5. Suppose others do their best and are willing to forgive when the situation arises. Training to forgive someone takes you a long way to show yourself how to forgive.

The above five points are an excellent way of reducing or removing all pressures in your life. Here are a few other things that you can do. Think of it as a bonus material-my reward in my article for having gone so far. A representative of new jobs tells no to prevent more obligations. Learn to ignore the criticism of others often. Jogging is another great way to reduce your life's tension, whether you have time to ponder the issues of life or time to escape for a while.

Another way to reduce stress is to take a holiday. Holidays are holidays to get away from the usual busy times and for a week or two to take a different view. But be careful. Don't want to do too much on your holiday and map it all out. If you do, the time you have planned to relax becomes work. When you try to cramp too much on your holiday, keeping up with schedules and deadlines never works. It will only lead to more stress, the very thing that you are trying to avoid ironically.

Stress can also be reduced by simple respiratory exercises wherever you are.

Attract through the nose, hold on, and exhale your mouth for 5 seconds. Repeat the process ten times, and you will feel the release of stress and tension and concentrate on your breath. The slow inhalation of oxygen will not only make you feel better, but you will experience stress release when you exhale. Activities like breathing and meditation allow you to focus your attention for a short time elsewhere. Meditation and stress management exercises return the body to a relaxed state, enable it to heal itself, and avoid damage. The physical effects of meditation on our bodies reduce our heart rate and slows our respiration.

One approach some people should consider is aromatherapy to help reduce tension and feel better. The purpose of aromatherapy is to have beneficial effects on the scents of these essential oils. Stress relief doesn't mean escaping stress; it's all about taking it into account. Meditation teaches the vital ability to live in the present for 15 to 20 minutes. Yet awareness skills help you to live an optimistic life every day, as tension has been seen is part of life. Not all pressure can be avoided or should be avoided. Knowing how to know when too many things crowd into life and saying no in time is one of the best things you can do for yourself and for the people you care about. If you see someone you believe to be overwhelmed today, put them aside, and warn them against the physical and emotional dangers of such a course. You should teach them about deep breathing and meditation. All this helps you build psychological and physiological defenses against future stress. But this isn't a one-time fix. Be vigilant of potential tension rises. To experience these things early on means that you control your own life more. One important thing is to maintain the right balance in your physical, spiritual, and emotional growth. Do these things, and not only will you be healthier, but you will also be happier.

The Difference Between Visualization and Meditation As a Method For Reducing Stress

Many people think visualization is the same as meditation, but not. There are similarities, but also a big difference between the two. Meditation aims to separate oneself from the thoughts, while visualization includes the imagination and is more involved. The confusion comes from modern marketing, which provides reflections to many directed imagery items. Let's look at both approaches.

There are several ways to meditate. Conscious breathing is one of the simplest. The best way to relax is to lay down or sit in a comfortable chair. Make sure that your chest and diaphragm have enough space to expand as you breathe.

Start by observing your breathing–don't control it; just feel it. Consciousness alone can slow it down. There'll be other thoughts; let them float away. Take your attention back to your breath. The goal is to keep the focus passive.

Then try breathing into your nose for a count of 5, later out into your mouth for a count of 5. Don't push it, just let it happen. Just make it happen. Feel the air flowing through your nose and your lips. Let the air pass to all parts of your body, accumulating anxiety and tension that can then be relieved. The next step brings peace and relaxation. Continue this 20-30-minute practice, or as long as you can comfortably.

Do not be discouraged if unwelcome thoughts hit you! With practice, you can automatically let them slide out when they enter.

It's like a holiday in your mind to imagine a peaceful scene. If you feel stressed, you can do that! The next time you are in a stressful situation, find a quiet place to lie on a tropical beach for a few minutes, close your eyes, and imagine. Feel the sand under your body; the sun warms your skin, the touch of your hair. Breathe profoundly and welcome the feeling of complete relaxation in your body. A few minutes from this will induce the calming response of your body, because your mind can not tell the difference between real and imagined things!

Whatever method you choose is a personal matter of preference. If you do something to help your mind get away with anxiety, you're on the right path. And you will feel happier, comfortable, and refreshed at the end of your visualization.

CHAPTER THREE:
PROTECT AND RENEW YOUR SPIRIT DURING THE HOLIDAY SEASON!

The holidays are a time for happiness and joy for many of us. Supportive family and friends often surround us. What an unforgettable gift. If this is your case, you probably do not need much protection during your holidays, and your spirits are probably refreshed by gathering these supporters. Though this is not the case for many of us. Therefore, it is essential to consider how you get with more motivation and satisfaction than discouragement and sadness through this holiday season.

Once you speak about preserving and renewing your spirit, it needs to be clear what it means by talking about your vision. How do you explain your mind? Spirit is described as the "essential nature of one's person;' the fundamental concept or animating force within the living beings;’ “incorporate consciousness." What does this mean for you? How would you characterize your spirit? You can hear someone saying, "she has such a strong spirit."

One of the first things you can enjoy all year round and during your holidays is to be surrounded by people who accept you and your account. Once, perhaps these are the types of people you'll be around during the holiday season. What a blessing, if so! But if you don't like the people with whom you spend the holidays, then encourage you to saturate with those who accept you before the holidays or trips. Adapt these people to your timetable, whether this means having a dinner date with them before you travel or before the event. Or maybe it is to stay in contact with them while you or they are away by telephone, email, or text. It is essential to remain linked to your inner self, your spirit.

Let's assume, for starters, that you are a very spiritual person, open-minded. Perhaps you are equal in your opinion and enjoy very insightful conversations. Most of your close friends have the same viewpoint and love your way of thinking and embrace it. But the family in which you married is very conservative and has limited views on different subjects. Over the years, you know that in your conversations, you can only be superficial without causing friction in the family. So, while you can enjoy your family at the level you know how to do, it is vital to be nurtured by those who can speak and understand and embrace your language. You don't have to open to those who only stomp around you and don't accept your differences.

It is equally important to be as prepared as possible for what you might face during your vacation with those who support you. One way to do this is to extend the site! Know what you're going to get into. Be informed and be responsible. Will this be an environment more secure than not? Many conditions (like families) are often encountered, to understand the dynamics enough to know what to expect. Many circumstances are fresh, so you can do your best to understand how the opportunity will be. For example, if you are invited for the first time to a neighborhood party or a working party. This is a new experience. However, general information can be gathered. You may ask other people who were there what the parties are usually like. You might find, for instance, that the work party is very formal, and everyone is well kept. Or the neighborhood party is a just gathering for adults and drinks where many of you wake up with bad gossip. You may not want to attend a neighborhood party when you are a newly recovering alcoholic, or you may want to bring some non-alcohol drinks.

Dress for the occasion, finally! If you go somewhere, that feels very safe and agrees, go for it! Wear your best and most fun and comfortable outfit or dress, whatever you are. If there are threats or if your souls are dangerous, wear your protective gear! Don't let anything hang out. It's your job to keep you safe and protect yourself.

The holiday spice is a great time to regenerate your mind. It's so easy to get caught up in all the excitement of the season that you can burn up. What do you think about renewing the word? A general definition of renewal is "to make new or as new," as defined in the online TheFreeDictionary. I urge you to follow the Five "Rs": restore, rebuild, restart, reaffirm, and fill in. Each of these is closely linked, but each has a different dimension.

To restore means to "make new or as if new; to return to or to a former or original state." Several factors of life may cause some of our vital resources to get dull or buried. Perhaps you were in an abusive relationship and just recently got rid of that. You are invited to think about any qualities that may have to be brought back to the forefront of your life. Perhaps your partner did not like yourself to spend time with others, so you squashed that social part of yourself. Part of your restoration can return to socialization and get people around.

Reviving means "reviving or thriving, returning to consciousness or life." What part of your fundamental self could have to be restored? Are you creative and artistic, but did you tuck this part away? Are you caught up in the everyday system and all its demands and lost your spontaneous and adventurous sides? You can sometimes be so severe that you forget to play.

Resume means "return to or start again after interruption; return to yourself." It's very similar to the two above, but you hope everyone will help to spark different ideas. It brings up my issues for me for starters. For many years my spiritual life was so to speak on the back burner for various reasons. Then you started to focus on and analyze that aspect of my life and began to assert that essential part of myself.

Reaffirm. Remember. Affirm means "to affirm as valid or confirmed." It would assert something of significance within ourselves again or again. My creative side is an example of this for me. You were so fascinated with children and my clinical practice and all the projects that you didn't support other innovative needs in your life. Starting writing articles and my book was an excellent example of how I reaffirmed this essential part of my life. This part of me makes me feel alive, and you're less effective in other areas without it.

Replenishing means "filling with inspiration or power; filling up or rebuilding." Why can't you use a refill? What a better time than the holiday season to participate in activities that inspire and empower you! What happens to each of us is different. Maybe what will fill you up is a spiritual meditation weekend retreat. Or perhaps an evening with your long-standing girlfriends. The gift of replenishing your spirits seems to be at the top of your holiday list.

With a little attention to your needs, during this holiday season, you can protect and renew your spirits. It is within your power to track your focus and behavior and to ensure that you take care of your needs. This time of year, is a beautiful experience of holiday cheer. The more helped you are, the more you can get to build a fun and enjoyable holiday season!

Relax, Renew and Restore Your Spirit with a Wellness Vacation

Wellness holiday? Sure, all of us need one.

Americans are busier than ever before. It's almost impossible to get out of our hustle and bustle with modern technology such as laptops and cell phones. Nevertheless, this intense, busy pace is why everyone needs a chance to enjoy a wellness holiday fully. The idea to spend one- or two-weeks practicing yoga or eating organic food is reasonably new but increasingly popular.

What's your ideal relaxing idea?

What would you think of as the most relaxing thing? Want to go on a sandy beach and feel the warm sand in your toes? Perhaps you want to climb a mountain or lie around a swimming pool. Regardless of the type of wellness package that you choose, the aim is to renew the spirit and come back home relaxing and rejuvenated, ready to face the stressful world of work and to pay the bills and get children to play football.

Stick to the most relaxing thing you've ever done for ten minutes. Do you not feel less anxious than to worry about it? Perhaps it is time to relax for a wellness holiday.

Why a healthy holiday?

Relaxation is one of the primary keys to good health. Those who meditate and practice yoga better sleep and feel good about life every day. Relaxation boosts your immune system and makes you less susceptible to diseases like hypertension and heart disease. A week or two away from everyday pressures can make a difference in your health and happiness.

A wellness holiday can help to create balance and harmony throughout the year. It can inspire you to relax more frequently.

Wellness holidays can be adapted to your personal needs and interests.

There are as many kinds of wellness holidays as well as well-being tourists. In two weeks, you can go to some exotic places such as Hawaii or Aruba or have a day or a weekend to enjoy massages, yoga classes or facials.

Freedom and the Spirit-Born Believer

Part One: Sphere of Liberty of the Holy Spirit You can not fully appreciate what Jesus Christ has done for us receptively without knowing first and foremost one of the main reasons for human creation. God loves liberty!

And freedom is a quality that God exercises when he wants to do and does something-" Our Lord is in the heavens, and He does as He intends... I know that you can do anything, and no intention of Yours can be thwarted "(Psalm 115:3 NIV; Job 42:2 ESV)- Adam was made to represent two attributes which are highly appraised by God, the freedom, in a world of liberty; Trust freely exercised and love openly expressed. These two qualities can not exist without a sphere of freedom. God created animals, fish, etc. that occupy the earth of the world, but these animals are controlled by an innate instinct built into their essential nature. Adam was created, on the other hand, with the freedom to choose his conduct, which was in no way compelled or manipulated. It could decide if you would go in a loving relationship with God or abuse His liberty and not trust God's warning and act with a particular option of disobedience. "The Lord God ordered the man,' You are free to eat from every tree in the garden. Still, you must not eat of the knowledge of good and evil, because if you do, you will surely die (literal) God so respects the independence that this attribute within mankind demonstrates the image and essence of God in us. The first line of Adam: Weber's Third New International Dictionary defines freedom as:' Quality or status of freeness and ability or ability to act without unnecessary hurdles or restrictions.' God created Adam without unnecessary hindrances or restraint so that he could either make his personal choice to obey God through his free trust in the word of God and thus to express his love. And, through abuse of his rights, he may freely express his disobedience and freely exercise action against God.

And as you know, Adam abused his liberty by disobeying God, but since he and his posts were trapped in a sphere of sin, fault, and death-" Therefore as, by one man (Adam) came into the world in (a self-centered, self-pleasing life away from God and the things of God), and death by sin, so also death spread among all men because they all sinned "(Rom. 5:12 ESV) After Adam and Eve had misuse of liberty, but it is recorded in the Scriptures that his descendants were not born in the image and likeness of God, but in Adam's picture of sin and death–"This is the written account of the line of Adam (Heb: toledo;' yÄlad' means' to produce.' Once God created man, in the image of God, He created him. He created and blessed both male and female. He named them Man (Heb:' ÄdÄm, the personal name as well as the crown of the creation of God) when they were made. When Adam lived for 130 years, he had a son in his likeness, in his face, and he called him Seth, which is what Adam's likeness means in his descendants, and Adam died... Seth is gone... Enosh is gone... Kenan is dead... (Here is the beginning record of Adam's descendants in his likeness). "(Genesis 5) The historical record of

Adam's descendant who had been born in his likeness is one of sin and death, where the sphere of freedom was lost in the things of God! Another Man's lineage but wait a minute! (and the born spirit-believers) are formed in the likeness of God in true righteousness and holiness "(Romans 6:23 ESV; Ephesians 4:24b)-" Do not wonder that I told you," You must be born again; literally, you must be born from above, and the new spiritual creation comes from God and not man. Thus the Apostle John states to everyone born from the Holy Spirit that God's Spirit is the Source of a sinner's new birth— "Jesus came to himself (the creation), and His people (The Israelites) didn't receive Him. But to all who received Him, who simply believed," To the active and obedient trust) "in His Name, He gave them the right to be the children of God. He was separated from the Source of Life, and he lost the realm of freedom where the beauty, peace, and joy of God reign supreme. Because God values such high freedom, where love and trust can thrive, and because "we are rich in mercy, through the great love with which He loved us, even when, as Adam's descendants in our transgressions, we were saved (from the world of sin, guilt, and the judgment of death)... For by grace, you were saved.

Your connection with the death and resurrection of Christ occurs in the restoration of your soul by the Holy Spirit and puts you in the realm of God's great love and freedom.

Death becomes an open door: in Jesus Christ, we trust that when physical mortality takes our earthly bodies, we will go to the presence of our Lord and Savior Jesus Christ directly—"We believe yet we are pleased to be absent from our[earthly] body and present with him.

Favor From the Holy Spirit and the Three Anointing Levels

Who favors and unites and what is the object of salvation in these last days is a must? These give Christians the world's benefit. In the church, anointing is spray around a lot, and most Christians do not understand it.

If you were redeemed, you are at 1 of 3 levels. You are ungodly to owe something to someone else.

Anointing doesn't mean you're religious, super just, or super blessed. Understand what anointing means before you pray because you're going to pay a bill. When it comes to the anointing, there is nothing to me. The higher the degree to which you reconcile, the greater the responsibility you have to the Lord and others. The bigger your calling, the higher the problem God presents you for others to solve.

Isaiah 10:27 says their burden will lift from your shoulders that day, and their yok will be cut off from your necks because you've grown fat (in the spirit).

What Isaiah says here is that you are empowered to break oppression and yokes and the slavery of others. These are the things we will do in Christ's name. Unction is God's power to do something, to change things, and to accomplish the mission. It is a divine facilitator. It is when God puts his super on your flesh. You can do something that you can not do in your capacity and display that supernatural strength.

In the church, we hear great talk about unction, but very little evidence of supernatural ability. Today, we have more strength and discernment than people had in Acts two thousand years ago. Today, though, we see less evidence of it. Citizens should be able to see the results of the unction in their marriage, jobs, employment, kids, and church. If we ever understood the greatness of our God and the power which it was willing to give us, we never again dreamed of a little and we ran towards others and said: "Let me here give you some of this unlet in your life," the unlet comes from the Holy Spirit, who poured into our vessels through us with an overflow of power to touch others. It fulfills your life and fills your destiny. If your achievements are low, your salvation will be small. You will learn how to increase your degree of anointing in this book. There is a disparity between the baptism of water and the uncle. The baptism of the Holy Spirit is like being baptized into a new identity, into death if you want to live in another life in a spiritual realm.

The levels of the unction of the Holy Spirit are

1. Okay, level (born again or level of manna mosaics) This is where God provides you with nour, meets your needs while you're in spiritual milk. It's a miracle time when you have nothing, and God is opening all the doors to your new birth, leading to a new man, while the older man is dying. You stop looking for love, oh, taste, and see that it's right in all places. You begin by feeling a spring of your life, you only know not enough of his word to understand how it is happening, but you may feel alive for the first time or at least sometime before your spirit and joy were robbed from the sin of the world. The high level is the most significant testimony of the blood's strength.

2. River Level (a divine gift is demonstrated) This is the level of seed and harvest where confidence is no more in reach. Your Bethel, where your life falls to God, is called the river point. Now you live in the values of the Kingdom.

3. The degree of rebirth (empowerment or a double portion of Elijah's redemption, where you can call things that are not like manifesting them).

The Samaritan woman with Jesus at the well. He said to her; I'd have given it to you if you only understood the gift of God and had asked. You're never going to thirst again if you drink this water that I give you. It will be a water well that begins to burst (level 1 at conversion).

John 7:37, Let anyone who thirsts come and drink. I'll give you living water rivers flowing out of your belly. This is the Baptism of the Holy Spirit by the faithful. You have rivers of living water in the Baptism of the Holy Spirit and begin to work in the strength of the Holy Spirit. This is anointing level 2. Your well and river depend on the spiritual world in which you live. Are you fed the word? Are you spending time in prayer? Do you first put the Lord? Will you walk in the values of the Kingdom? Are you sowing seed? If your church has a low river, you can't go down the stream very well. Your catch in soul fishing (or other Christians maturing) will be small.

The first two levels are replaced by the third level, the main level. The live wire of the well and the river is Rain. Take away the Rain and the well, and the river is damaged. There are some activities you can do in the well and in the river, but you have to rain. If you have the water, then you can get the storm. Then you have control. Ask the Lord in the spring for the Rain, he is making the clouds of wind. He gives men showers of Rain, all plants of the ground. Ask, and He is going to provide you with anointing, particularly during the season God wants to bless you. So it is vital to know the seasons of God's blessings. We live in the latter holy house, and the redemption of God is upon the church, and we should begin to anticipate healings and good works.

Joel 2:23, O people of Zion, rejoice in the Lord thy God, for in righteousness the Rain of fall has brought thee. This sends plenty of showers both in the fall and in the spring. The Holy Spirit's power in the Rain comes in Adar (April) month and Tishrei month (October), Passover, and the Tabernacle festival. We're about the rainy season of the autumn anointing beginning in October at the Sukkot festival. At the same time, the power of the Holy Spirit came upon Mary as she conceived and supernaturally bore the Messiah. In these seasons, God wants to show His power and glory. I assume that in the season of the feast of tabernacles, the second coming of Christ will be. If you want your church to bursting forth with ungodly force, get your feet up and lift your voices to Him. Recall, said Jesus, if only you'd inquire.

In the church, there will be a strength as you never saw, as our Savior is about to gather His Bride. A supernatural rain will hit the church in Sukcot's (Tabernacles') season, so begin to search for the clouds, get ready, get ready for the Lord's souls in his season of blessings if you want to save the lost, plan for maturity.

One must scream because the Rain replaces what the devil has stolen, someone is returned to ill health, someone goes to another degree of unction. He will send you the promotion intended for you. He will show his glory in your midst. Don't sit back and lament over someone's onlooker, hop on their little coat, and get yourself rubbed on with some of those blessings. That's why they're salvaged to bless you, and you didn't even have to pay the cost for the anointing. Go down to the altar and let some of the ungodly pray and lay hands upon you.

God wants to restore families and to gain the strength of the Holy Spirit from churches. In the latter holy building, God will take some men from their feet and call and unclean them. The Bible says that you are going to eat plenty when the rain comes, and people are going to know that God is with you. Everyone wants what you have, and they're going to know that God is in your midst. Now I see hungry churches, and we see more prayer intercessory, anointing with oil and foot washing returned to many churches I visited. Don't fall asleep; keep your spiritual eye open for these manifestations in the church. In the past year or so, I have seen more gifts over service with priests, worshippers, encouragers, people with knowledge, and great discernment.

However, you see that the level of your salvation depends on the volume of the river and how many people you can transport. It's not "me," it depends on how many people you can bring down. It is about how many deposits in other lives you can produce. When you think it's all about you, you might forget that your levels are rising for the wrong reason. Let the "me" go, and God's going to fill you. The only reason you have been packed with uncleanness is that it overflows to the benefit of others. So those who walk around the church believing that they are the only ones to be salvaged are nothing else but a false witness, see and see if the manifestation suits them. Does your leadership bring souls? Do they help Christians mature? Will they take yokes and burdens away? Will they feed the word of God hungry and thirsty? Should they nurture the young Christian, help the widows and control the life of some child in the church? Do they call you in the hospital or when you're sick?

The Holy Spirit is not just words with POWER. Acts 4:8 Peter already filled with the Holy Spirit said, "Behold, you rulers of the earth, you are better to hold fast, for I come, and I am come strengthened. So now offer courage to your servant, Yahweh." And He reached out his arm and spoke courageously. That day, three thousand people were rescued.

Right now, Peter shows you what to do when your church level is low; fast, pray, and ask. Praise His holy name, then pray again and ask the Lord to give you a replenishment, so that you can enter your task. Church people don't have, because they don't inquire. They give up too quickly because there is no effort to pray. If there is no intercessory evening of prayer in your church, start one, as those powerful prayer sessions change things in your church and life and ensure that the Holy Spirit is present among yourselves.

When Jesus came out of the water after John had baptized him, the unlet rested in the shape of a dove upon him, and he was prepared to begin his work and fate. He loved the presence of God, and God had been with him. The Holy Spirit never left Jesus because the Holy Spirit was never grieved.

If the Holy Spirit grieves you, nothing is done, no redemption without anointing, that is why God wants to unclean you so severely. It only increases because of its use. When he sings and dances, when he speaks, then he teaches, if he prays, he is a prayer warrior, if he loves and worships and then the Holy Spirit reveals himself within himself and leads us out. If it lays its hands-on people, go down to the altar and lay hands on heavy people with yokes, fortresses, and plague. When he asks you to dance down the island, then take your shoes.

If your life does not produce results, then there is no unction. Don't come to church to act or to fill the "me," give us some results in your life and what you do in others. Get up on Sunday morning to go to church and bless someone else. Real Christians need not your actions. We know that the Holy Spirit is genuine now. It's not how you fall out at the altar; it's how you get up and do it. These are the things that the ungodly look at from you, not your cry. If you have a yell, you should also have fruit.

I know what you're thinking, well I'm going to say things as I move out into my unclean people. Okay, let them speak about you, but keep Christ's heart set. If people disagree with you or when a disaster arrives, you must remain ungodly when the doctor tells you to live for six months. And yeah, it costs to be immoral. It takes faith and brings God and not a man into your heart. It takes faith to step in and give your life for love and compassion because you don't want to sometimes, but you must sacrifice yourself every day to preserve your unction.

Could you miss your uncle? Ultimately, if you turn your attention off from Christ and on yourself or start to worry about your picture of man, or become pleasing people, you will be counterfeited. What you make is known to be falsified. By failing to pray, praise, and worship and not to live according to the principle of seed, you can lose your salvation. The quickest way to lose your life is by the tongue. The "me" thing, derogatory talk, funny gossip, rage and discord, arrogance and jealousy, sin or disobedience to God's call to your life. A prime example is King Saul.

The three ways to bring redemption to the physical realm from the spiritual realm:

1. Acts of justice

2. To walk in faith, to reveal the fruit of the spirit

3. Life of prayer and worship Don't wait for people to tell you whether you are ungodly; start walking in your unction, and people will see your experiences.

This book discusses who is anointed and why the Holy Spirit chose a person for a task and task. Also, you will see how to boost the degree of unction and how to focus on the people you have been inspired to meet by the Holy Spirit.

CHAPTER FOUR:
HOW TO RESTORE YOUR POWER TO CREATE

You have come to earth as a spirit with the power of the universe to do whatever you want. Your name was "I AM," and you are part of all that surrounded you since you were able to open your eyes. No crib, mother or father, brother or sister, walls, or ceilings were present. You've been them, and they've been you. While you had time and space with what you saw, you didn't understand that you weren't what you saw, felt, tasted, or heard. Even stinking diapers didn't have any significance for you. You didn't want or need anything, because it was outside your consciousness and experience.

Then something happened; you started communicating with your parents, and they began to educate you about the world. Every time someone came into the room—it was your name—

you eventually responded to a sound. You became "I am Roy" now, and you began to discover that in the new world, you had some personal power. But you did not always understand why you did not still get what you wanted, and people didn't always respond as you liked it.

As you grew older, people around you restricted your influence by asking you what you could and could not do or have, and the power you received into life was, of course, severely limited by that time. It would help if you were within limits set by your parents, your community, and your country. You received an inherited belief system or religion from your parents, the right legislation, and the right detergent to use from your grandmother.

Five words were given to you every day to disempower you, to kill the spirit, and become dependent on you. These words are "right and wrong," "good and bad," and the most disempowering of all "can't!" The only way to combat them was to violate their laws and turn them away, and to use their language. And because you always believe you are only the physical body, you are powerless to change the world, and God punishes you. You are unrelated to who you are and what you are. You don't know you're the creator and not the victim.

You are limited not only to those with power over you but also to a punishing God with control over your kin. You wouldn't get anything if you had to get down to your knees and beg for it more than likely, because you weren't worth it. You also had to support the institutions that taught you these things. Failure to comply would mean even less influence of your destiny in this or any other lifetime.

Time has shown that humanity is incapable of complying with systems, rules, or precepts designed to control humanity's spiritual nature. The system that removed our power is breaking down now.

In our time, religion accounts for around 84% of the world's population. It is a religion that led you to this point in your evolution and is the most significant influence on how you live today.

Religion is responsible for the highest part of what is happening in the world in our history; "social revolution," because you are so powerless that you feel that you are not making or are responsible for how you behave, whether intimate, worldly, or natural circumstances. God was the scapegoat and the convenience to take responsibility or accountability for yourself. Until recently, only a few who used it were aware of the extent of our power.

The longer you live it, the more your spiritual awareness develops slowly. It's because you bought what you are taught, and you don't see the need. But with age, wisdom comes to know what is and what might have been. At that point, many gave up and found it too much hassle or effort to change.

There is a sure way to do it one step at a time for those who have ever felt this way, and for those who want to take back their power.

It can easily be summarized in one phrase and explained; It's a simple, methodical technique that helps you to have your life and to know the power that you have always had to build wealth, good health, and happiness.

To do this, you must possess the circumstances of your life, all you do, and everything that others do for you and everything that comes naturally. You can't give what you don't possess.

You're one of two things; you're a victim or a builder. The exercise is to know yourself as your creator. Even the most illuminated would find this very idea challenging. But you must remember that your past dictates these thoughts. You must, therefore, take small steps to resolve them.

From now on, all that happens to you is a direct result of your desire, on certain levels of your awareness. Either good or bad works for you or not, it must be owned by you. You are the maker, and there is a cause. You build all your life circumstances. The scapegoat here may, therefore, be your subconscious so that you are not willing to own it at a higher level. It is not the will of God, and it is not that you are capable or incapable of natural circumstances, or you are at the right time in the wrong place. It's not that you're lucky or unlucky or that something has happened. Because can or can not be known to you now, everything is your creation. Even if you must lie to yourself for a while, you must possess everything you experience.

You must know that your duty is also injuries and sickness. You construct them at some level of consciousness for your reason. Take that responsibility; whether you like it or not and know it was for reasons made–don't give it away or blame anyone or anything. You will eventually be able to change or avoid these things by doing this. When you give up your control, you become a helpless victim and unable to change your circumstances. Do not try to outthink and ask yourself; why do I want to do this, why do I do it to myself or I can't do it. Accept your power to make them happen for whatever reason you know or don't know, and eventually, you will control them and turn them around. Remember, know that all things or situations are not "good" or "evil." Everything was created for your purpose, whatever it may be. In retrospect, you'll figure out the explanation.

It could be a good thing to drop a hammer on your big toe if it gets your awareness-it works for you. It may be an indication that in your life, something doesn't work; time to make a change. A trip to the doctor may give you the chance to meet your soul mate. It's for a reason, embrace your purpose, and you know the power to create your entire life situation. It's not the will of Allah, you are not a victim, and you manifest all the events of your life.

Consider your control no longer in every moment of your life from this point on. Don't listen to the old thoughts; create new ideas. Tell yourself in every minute of every day that you are the creator; that whatever you do is to your purpose. Whatever other people may say or do; you don't give up your power. It can be slow and painful, but it does work. Build this knowledge inside you, and you will be the person you always thought you were. You're never going to be a victim again.

Remember, it never works in your favor, regardless of the circumstances. Even if someone has physical power over you at this stage, realize that you created a situation for your sake at some level, hold on that thought, and you will, at some point, have the power to change it. Most significantly, as you understand your ability to create, you will no longer need unwelcome interactions to lead you to things that don't work in your lives.

Avoid judgment, because you will fail, even in judging your own experiences.

So, if the boss calls you today and fires you, you did it for a higher purpose. It wasn't luck or chance, should you win the lotto; it was your ambition, your determination that made it happen. For your larger purpose, all things work. And whether you believe it or not, you have the power to change them. This exercise helps you get to know your strengths. Recognize the doubt and understand that it is natural to happen, to possess the doubt, and to give it away. It's your doubt, nobody else, and you've got the power to get over it. The quick you work on it, the more it will manifest itself in your life.

Restoration of the Dominion Image of God in Man

We also search for glory and legitimacy in this life because we must realize that it is for this reason; it is God who created us. There was a conversation when God started to develop people. Then God said, "Let us make man, as we are, after our image, and let them rule over the fish of the sea, over the birds of the air, and the flocks, upon all the earth, and upon all the creeping things which creep upon the earth." God created man, then, in His very image, created him, both men and women. So God blessed them, yet God said, "Fulfill the world, and multiply it; and make the earth whole, and subdue it, and rule over the fish of the sea, and the birds of the air, and over all that moves on the earth." Gen 1:26-28. Here we see that in His image, God planned to make us. Where we are not yet sure of the origin and meaning of the image of God, God Himself describes His creation, "In Our image, in

Our likeness, let them reign over the sea... the air and the earth." We can call this image or express it as "the dominion-image of God."

The Hebrew word for dominion is' Radha'[pronounced rä·dä] which means 1) to rule and dominate, and to dominate (overlook), to tread (a) (Qal) to be ruler, to rule and to subjugate (b) (Hiphil) to have dominion and (2). The concept of the sovereignty of God is that the heart within us that instinctively seeks to reign over the environment we live in. The' dominion image' is also the legal right to rule the world as God rules the whole universe. This verified by the Bible, "The Lord [i.e., under His dominion] is the heaven, even the heavens, but the earth He has given to the people" (Ps 115:16).

Nevertheless, the issue is that the concept of the sovereignty of God will only be real if the man is associated with God in the Spirit. Because God did not speak in singularity, but in plurality, while thinking about His image[i.e. He did not say,' I will make man in My image,' but he said,' Let us make man in Our image{ which includes the Father, the Son, and the Holy Spirit}.' God's strength lies in the role played by every person in the trinity to communicate His creative image of leadership that He exercises over His law. Therefore, God is three in person, but one in purpose. This is clear implies that unless the human being relates to God in his Spirit with one mission, he can not express this image of God in his life. Trinity's power lies in its unity. This unity can be described as a dependency on one another and a spiritual connection between each other. The Bible says, "The Spirit now is the Lord" (2 Cor 3:17). In other words, the Lord is now bound by this time-space, this Earth's domain [i.e., The relation of God on this Earth] is the Holy Spirit human. It also means that the Holy Spirit acts in us as the Lord over us and in this world through us. This dependence on God the Spirit activates the image of God's dominion in us. The vision of the supremacy of God would give us a unique identity and prominence by restoring God's original purpose in us. In other words, we are engineered and designed exclusively to achieve this goal. Praise the Lord! Praise the Lord!

His picture of dominion, God created man that He might exercise authority just like Him. Jesus was the one who showed the exact image of God on this planet earth the first time Adam lost in disobedience (1 Cor 15:45,49; Luke 3:38). For example, when Jesus exercised domination upon Earth, he told the hypocritical religious leaders who opposed Him, "If I cast out demons through the Spirit of God, surely the kingdom of God has come upon you" (Matt 12:28). In other words, Jesus told them that the Divine picture of God is what the Spirit of God himself performs. In opposing the works of the Spirit of God who worked in Jesus, these people were already against the reign of God who came upon the Earth through Jesus, which the Pharisees boasted as the true representatives. In the following verses, he spoke of his erroneous critical and judicial attitude in attributing the Spirit's work to Satan's work, which can\not is forgiven forever as these religious persons have wished to break God's purpose to exercise the image of God in the world (Matt 12:31-32). Jesus represented all of us to God, and he is the "repairer of the breach" (Is 58:12), or the repairer of a humankind's lost God connection.

Jesus also reiterated this expression of God's concept of superiority when He commented, "I assure you, the Son can do not anything of Himself, but what He sees the Father doing: for whatever He does, the Son is doing in the same way as He does." For the Father who loves the Son, and He is showing Him all that Himself does, and He will teach Him more works than these, to marvel "(John 1:2). Jesus also said,"... the Father that abides in Me worketh" (John 14:10). In other words, the works of Christ on this planet earth were equivalent to the work of the Father, God Himself residing on this earthly body and doing His jobs on Earth because of his spiritual connection with God the Father. This spiritual connection with God by the Holy Spirit brings the image of God to rule in us and to reign in this world

(Eph 2:18). The power to rule and rule on this planet Earth is equivalent to the flow of communication between God and us. The more connected we are with God to represent God in His likeness, the higher the power of authority on this Earth and the image of God's rule.

The more we express it, the better and more unique our identity in God will be. This is the place where God's enemies in the world of Spirit will come to recognize God's dominion image in and through us, just as the wicked Spirit confessed himself when he rebounded and attacked seven faithless sons of Sceva, a Jewish priest without any God-connection. God's dominion-image] within them, in their spiritual man (Acts 19:13-15). As the Bible states in Acts 19:15-16, "And the evil spirit answered, saying,' I know Jesus, and I know Paul, but who are you? "And the man in whom the evil Spirit was spring upon them has overpowered and dominated them, and they fled naked and wounded from that house." Only when in your spiritual man, you are firm and have a mature image of God within you, will all principalities and powers know you and recognize in you the power of God.

Once Adam disobeyed God, the sovereignty image of God was lost. The rule of the world remained in Adam's hand until the day when "sin came into the world" (Rom 5:12). When we inquire about what is sin? What is sin? The Bible says, "La wretchedness is sin" (1 John 3:4). In other words, sin is the lawless existence of the devil, who continually works against and fights against the rule of God (1 John 3:8). As Satan's criminal life legitimately affected human beings through Adam's disobedience, they became all sinners through our inborn soul (Rom 5:19). Adam's spiritual connection with God was just dead on the day Just as God had warned Adam of his disobedience (Gen 2:16-17), Satan began to use his voice, after Adam's intimate relationship with God was broken up, to guide man to the soul, as God created the soul to be operative in spiritual direction. Jesus reiterated this fact by stating that Satan's voices and demons, identified by him as "the voice of strangers," are rejected by the believer (John 10:5). The more people are deceived by the voices of these spirits in their soulish realm, the more lawless they become. But the faithful will listen to the real voice of God because of God's brand-new soul to connect to him (Ezek 36:26-27). Such believers must begin to hear God's voice, and He will also call them by name and guide them, as He has promised (John 10:3-4). The Spirit of God will connect the voice of God directly from his heavenly throne to our earthly soul. Through our enabled Spirit, our soul will hear God's voice on earth (1 John 3:24; Heb 12:25; 1 Cor 2:10-12).

Thus, the supremacy of man on earth is closely linked to his dependence and association with God through his soul, which is only relived, regenerated, and renewed for a born-again believer in Christ Jesus (Eph 3:16; Tit 3:5; 2 Cor 4:16). Therefore, Jesus alone says, "I tell you most surely, except a man be born with water or of the Spirit, he can not enter into the Kingdom of God.

The things that are born the flesh are flesh, and the things that are born of the Spirit are Spirit." In other words, Jesus says that the Spirit of God alone can bind a person's dead Spirit to the everlasting existence of God's kingdom. Only the voice of the wind, which is God's Holy Spirit, is heard by the born from above (John 3:8).

The reason many people are more oppressed than ever before is because they don't accept God's truth and receive it[i.e., The Holy Spirit] loves Jesus and His voice; they love to hear and receive misleading, soulful words that are contrary to the truth of God expressed in the name of God (John 8:32; 2 Thessalonians 2:9-12). 2 Cor 4:4, the Apostle Paul clearly states these things in his writing, "the thoughts of the god of this age, who believe not, are blinded, lest the light of the evangelized glory of Christ shine upon them, who is the image of God." The dominion image of God shines upon us as much as we believe to receive the light of the glorious gospel of Christ. Until a man has a hunger to hear and receive the truth, he can never distinguish between the voice of God and the soulful voices he can listen to in himself. That is why humans can not govern and rule this planet earth. Satan and his evil counterpart tyrannically control them and invisibly rule the world by spreading chaos, death, and pacification on the planet. Satan was able to blind the minds of the people and deceive them, because without God man has no power to rule. Man is wired that the only way he will rule the world is by his harmony of mind, soul, and body with God (Luke 1:37). Jesus humbly confessed this fact by saying, "I can do nothing of Me..." even though it was God's only begotten Son who came from heaven to this planet earth as the perfect incarnate substitute for every human being (John 5:30; 3:16,17).

Satan and his evil associates are much more potent than men as spiritual beings when the Spirit of God does not interact with him. Instead, the Apostle John wrote to the faithful, with divine inspiration: "You are of God, little ones, and overcome; for he who is in you[i.e., the Holy Ghost of God] is more than he who is in the world (i.e., Satan this and his demons)" (1 John 4:4). In other words, in his spirit-man, man is greater than Satan and all his wicked demons. also confirmed in Ps 8:5-6: "For you made him a little lower than the angels [i.e., Elohim.heb-> God Creator], and have crowned him with glory and honor. You made him dominate over the works of Your hands. You have [already] brought all things under his feet[including the angels]..." However, the Jewish tradition mistakenly translated it according to its culture and called God Angels simply because the word was pluralistic. But Christians do not have any trouble interpreting the Trinitarian doctrine as God the Creator in a diversified manner.]

Here we notice three things in the preceding verses,

1) By God's purpose, in man's original creation, man is only a small thing lower than God the Creator.

2) The very purpose of making man is to have control over him.

3) God has brought under His feet all things [i.e., Jesus Christ's feet] and sat us, humans, in the heavenly places with Him. By this high standing, we [i.e., The more significant than the angels are those who believe in Christ Jesus (Eph. 1:18-23; 2:5-6). So, only the New Testament angels in Heb 1:14 are accurately described as: "Therefore the angels are servant-spirits only sent to care for the people who inherit salvation." This was confirmed by an angel himself who said, "Be sure not to do so (i.e., to worship me): for I am thy fellow servant, and of thy brethren the prophets, and those who keep the words of this book, worshiping God" (Rev 22:9), when John's Apostle overwhelmed the prophetic words and views that came from the angel at the appointed time, he fell to adore the angel.

The original purpose and intention of God for man in His original creation is to be close to God and powerful with the image of God. This is His will for every man on earth on this planet (Romans 16:20). Satan didn't like God's proposal for him to be a human protector under him. He thus rebelled against God's planet earth mission. This is why Jesus taught His disciples to pray, "Your kingdom come, as in the heaven, you will be done upon the earth" (Matt. 6:10) since Satan has a rebellion against God, and since the fall of first Adam has instilled and influenced men to wrest God. Only the will of God on earth is not done because of the evil influence of Satan over all men on this earth.

By the intent of God's creation, people are designed to exercise dominance by relying on God and being in love. Only then will human beings have perfect peace, love, and unity for the practice of God's sovereignty on earth. Alone this will give prominence and identity to all people. Are you ready? Are you ready? You ask me what? What? Get this relationship with God right, and you will feel the picture of sovereignty of God within and through you. Praise the Lord! Praise the Lord!

Plant Spirit Shamanism - Soul Retrieval Through Nature

Shamans believe that pain, violence, shock-and essentially a dishonor of nature or a lack of connection may cause the soul to be lost.

There are still roadside shrines in many shamanic countries where people can relax, pay their respects to the natural world, and get cured and refilled.

Few such sacred places or rituals are remaining in the modern West. Festivals like May Day, originally the celebration of rebirth to celebrate the arrival of Spring, lost a good deal of their purpose and meaning. In turn, our souls, both individually and collectively, are weak, and many traditional societies regard us as the poorest people on earth, despite our great wealth and' power.'

Healing loss of soul often involves the shaman reconnecting his patient to nature, as you might feel from it, thus restoring balance and restoring the safe, healthy, and whole Spirit.

One approach in Japan is to accompany (or advise) the patient to walk into nature to meet a particular tree. Then she sits with her back and thinks about her troubles and sorrows in the forest.

As she listens carefully, the tree's Spirit— the magnificent gateway to nature— will tell her what to do while simultaneously taking and changing her pains, bringing her power and a new spirit back.

In Tuva, the patient will be advised to take a similar journey and give a natural shrine, where the spirits carry their soul back.

In both cases, the patient is naturally deeply immersed for nature, with the trees, and held in a quiet, revitalizing, and restful atmosphere in the woods.

In the Andes, healing of souls is a similar activity, but slightly different. Here, the shaman accompanies the patient to the physical location where the soul has lost its energy. The physical location is always the place of trauma, whether it's an accident blackspot where a car crash occurred or a house in the middle of childhood abuse. The soul is always locked in that place.

The shaman can bring the soul back by negotiating with the Spirit of this place and by attracting the soul to return by the singing of the joys that await the patient's body after the trauma is over. The shaman may make an offering in return for the soul in negotiations with the Spirit of place or leave flowers. When nature's spirits are pleased with the offer and assured that the soul they protect would be well served on their return-and if the soul itself feels loved and safe-they will be released to the patient immediately.

For example, when a child suddenly falls, his soul will leave his body and get ill. If this happens, an offering is made to heal the child instead of fall.

There are numerous ways to "call the soul." You can take a piece of your child's clothes and make a little doll and decorate with flowers or whatever the child likes and call his soul at the scared spot. You can also call and use the energies of plants, dove nests, feathers, tobacco, coca, or anything else necessary to help with this healing, but first ask Pachamama, the Spirit of the universe, before any session.

If the issue doesn't start in a fixed place, you go to the highest mountain or nearest river and carry out the ritual.

Across countries as diverse as Mexico, Haiti, and Peru, there is an alternative approach to soul retrieval, which also works with flowers. In these traditions, the soul can sometimes be not lost, but loosely attached, and at the same time vibrate in and out of the body. This can be done as a result of shock when events shaking your worldviews and undermine everything you thought right could also shake your mind. It's like you don't have anything to hold on, and your balance is gone. Such shocks may cause trauma, but if the soul is captured quickly enough, it can be cured before more profound wounding happens by forcing it back into the body and stabilizing it to restore balance.

One strategy is to cover the patient tightly into sheets or blankets to hold the soul back in the body. This may also be the cause of swaddling children, conventional persons understanding that a baby's soul is less attached to the physical organ of the baby and must remain so long as the child' grows into himself' and is formed in his body. The flower petals are placed inside the blanket and may also be rubbed on and around the patient.

When the patient lies in her sweet-smelling cocoon of flowers that calms the Spirit, the shaman sings to her with lullabies about the beauty of the world and how her people love and want it. Perfumes can also be sprayed on her; her aromas anchor her memory of the sweet words she hears and prayers for her soul and nature's spirits. So, she remains in the gentle warmth of the rising sun for a while before she is wrapped up and embraced as an initiation into a new way of life: a rebirth by flowers.

It grasps your mind and sends you off... before you hit the hurt spot. She faces you with pain. She heals the pain." Mexican teachings: Ceremonial Plant Spirits]. It parallels the Amazonian use of the cheap to remove negative forces and restore the patient's Spirit. In both cases, it is the plants that offer to heal directly. Interestingly, it is also feverfew that has long been respected for their healing and purification properties and is widely planted in ancient England in the belief that it purifies the air and prevents the spread of the plague.

Plant Spirit Shamanism believes that plants have a bond with human beings, know our suffering, and hope to love and heal. Just being close to them and their energy fields can suffice to call the soul back.

CHAPTER FIVE:
DEEP RELAXATION - LET YOUR SENSES GUIDE YOU

Most people generally recognize the five primary senses of vision, hearing, taste, smell, and touch. Although the way the body works is simplistic, it is crucial to group the main ways in which it's felt.

You may achieve a state of total relaxation by helping to consistently relax every sense and then linking the experience between each knowledge. - minds can independently reduce stress, but when all senses are relaxed, the results are so much higher.

It is best to put your focus elsewhere (like driving or caring for children) into a relaxed position like sitting or lying. I would recommend setting the alarm, so you don't have to check the clock, and if you wish, you can even go to sleep.

Relaxation by sight

For most people, the view is the primary concept. So, relax first for maximum effect. The eyes are uncomfortable and frustrating every day. You can rest by closing and placing a simple cold compress (some people use cucumber slices) or perhaps cotton wool moistened with a small amount of cold water.

Relaxation by Hearing

Relaxation when listening to certain sounds has a substantial impact on our minds and physiology. Most people have a song that makes them feel like taping or dancing their feet or making them glad or reflective when they hear it.

Human beings have a powerful sound affinity. Music is thought to have followed even cave paintings as a form of expression (as rhythmic drumming).

Finding compelling relaxation music at an appropriate rhythm to match your restful heart rate—this can be around 60 beats per minute for many. Combine it with spoken word techniques such as mediation or controlled imagery, and you have a compelling way to relax.

Relaxation by Taste

Many people find comfort food a great way to relax, but often the food you want is high in fat or salt and can make you uncomfortable.

One of the easiest ways to relax is to clean our palate (to regenerate our sense of taste) with a light (milk-free) infusion of your favorite tea, preferably decaffeinated as Camomile or Rooibus, at warm but not hot temperatures.

Relaxation by Smell

Fresh lavender can be very relaxing. Relaxing. Once you unwind, putting it next to a pillow can further improve your deep relaxation.

Relaxation with Touch

Head massage can help relieve muscle tension in the jaw and neck. Start from the back of the head and massage from the top of the neck in slow circles. Repeat several times with larger slow circles, which differ between medium and very light pressure.

A gentle pressure on the point that your jaw meets the skull just under and behind your cheekbones with the tips of the first three fingers on each side. Roll your fingers back and forth along the joint with very light pressure, and then slow down to your chin with a sweeping step.

The final and most crucial stage (forgetful of many)

Acknowledges the benefit of the process of relaxation. It is not enough to relax once you have time in your diary to regularly release your stress and accept this luxurious feeling of deep relaxation. Obtaining a tremendous profound relaxation CD can be an excellent way to avoid distractions. It is so easy to set time for relaxation. Please put it in your diary, starting perhaps for 10 or 15 minutes once or twice a week, and work towards a daily relaxation session when the expertise is better.

Simple Relaxation Tips

You walk through the times of your day, week, and month, and wish that you can relax for a while. It would appreciate fifteen or even ten minutes.

Just if you did not know, relaxation helps your body to re-energize; usually, the problem is that you are so intrigued and occupied with your' routine' that you don't have the time to relax or forget to take it.

Well, lucky to you, you read this because there are simple ways to relax comfortably, even during your busiest days. Simple and easy methods

Here are easy and straightforward Relieving Tips:

For those times at work: Often, you risk getting into trouble if you find yourself "relaxed." Nevertheless, there are some techniques that you can make while working that help to create a sense of calmness and will not be too much for others.

If you must sit on a computer all day, make sure you get up and move around every hour for a few minutes. It helps your body circulate blood. Just by changing the blood flow, you felt more alert and concentrated.

Roll your head around, from one side to side, front to back with your eyes closed while sitting at your desk. This technique helps to relieve tension in your neck and to increase the flow of blood to your brain. Also, roll your shoulders back a few times and then pull them out of your neck again a few times.

If you're on your feet all day long, stretch back and side, standing on the floor firmly, shoulder-width apart, and twisting from side to side slowly your upper body, including your head. This loosens your back and back muscles and releases tension throughout your body. A great tip is to stretch slowly with your hand out for the first time, so you can see how far you have spread. Close your eyes now and visualize yourself a bit further. Then open your eyes and stretch again, you will be surprised to find that you are doing a little more.

Go for a stroll during a break or lunch. Walking is a great way to clear your mind, and the extra exercise will also benefit your body.

During shopping: Rather than concentrate on the negative, as you believe there are not enough cashiers, all lines are 5 + deep, each with carts full of things to buy, take a deep breath, and relax your body.

Deep breathing helps to increase your blood oxygen. Your blood circulates the extra oxygen in your entire body to help recharge your internal systems.

The trick is to take five slow deep breaths. The right technique is to breathe and exhale your nose and mouth deeply.

It will not only help you relax with deep breathing; it will help to clear your mind, reduce brain fog, and make you feel much more alert and prepared to deal with your next platform project.

Deep breathing can be done everywhere if you feel stressed, or if you just want to clear your mind.

It is also better to count the breath and then count the breath. By pressing your thumb on each finger-

while inhale

1 (tapping rose)

 2 (tapping ring finger)

3 (tapping middle finger)

4 (tapping finger index)

Then exhale

1 (tapping index finger)

2 (drawing middle finger)

3 (topping ring finger)

 4 (tapping rose finger) repeat. This helps stretch your breath and turns your focus on your fingers from the outside world.

During the whole day: pause for a few moments and dream and let the hectic shackles of the world escape-dream like a kid in the evening before Christmas (or any day your inner child will dream the biggest).

Daydreaming releases your imagination, allows it to flow, which causes immediate relief from the inner stress of the' real' world.

Think of a place or experience which makes you feel comfortable or calm. Think of how it smells, how the air feels, and who's there. Don't take it lightly; our minds treat our active mental images as real-let your account create that picture for you... Feel the warm air breath, rip your t-shirt and hair, smell the aromas around you whether they are cookies or the ocean as the waves crash.

You will find that you feel relaxed, reinvigorated, and even ready to confront the real world with a much better view and attitude after about five minutes of a soothing daydream.

For EVERYWHERE, smile: Smile has shown itself to help you relax and rejuvenate your body.

Smile at others around you when you're out and around.

Smile at your friends when you are at work. It will not only help you relax, but it will also help you to relax.

Smile at your kids as you drive them around for all their various activities. This creates a peaceful environment for everyone to enjoy. You will find that they will smile back when you sincerely smile at them. What more relaxing heartwarming can you imagine a child smiling at you?

For if it is hard, laugh this is the next step from a smile (offensively) the laugh has also demonstrated to be an immediate stress reliever. Now it's quite sure you wouldn't want to be considered as a nut case (like the stalker smile in the above), so it might not be the most convenient time to laugh loudly when you are in line or sit at the desk.

Hypnosis for Relaxation and Stress Relief - Progressive Relaxation

Welcome to your ride to a better place. When you relax deep in your subconscious, you will get a chance to change the position that creates you every day again. Here suggestions come at the very heart of your being and become beautiful realities.

Central Part Follow this book to lead you to the depths of wellness, where you can fully revitalize your body and mind to precisely what kind of person you want to be living as you wish.

Let's continue. Let's start, close your eyes, relax your mind. Feel how your eyelids are like two moist, snug bodies, breathing each other's love. Now feel more and better the connection between them. Notice how one lid relaxes each pore, expanding gently towards the other, filling it with its cells with each small gap.

Allow yourself the chance to believe this. Your tightly paired eyelids cannot be forced apart. Open your eyes now. Feel like your eyelids don't just want to give up their relation if you try to stretch it out and isolate it. Now, close your eyes again and experience the perfect snugness they relax. Notice how the deep sense of calm sinks into your entire body and makes it bulky and relaxed. Experience the comfort of your body. Let it sink under you in the cushions. Imagine it giving a big, tired sigh as it falls into the pillows.

Let your consciousness travel to your forehead quickly. This is your imagination, and you're going to use it now. You look at a whiteboard. You've got a black pen printed on it in thick, smooth lines. Use the pen to draw a board circle. See your perfect circle. Outline an X. Take the eraser from the little rack on the whiteboard and delete the X. First, wipe out the ring. First, wipe out the entire situation and move deeper into peace and relaxation.

Focus on the point between your eyebrows from here. Combine all your attention in this position, guide your subconscious is entirely focused on the voice that you hear. Relax in space and listen to this voice as you relax deeper with every word. In the end, you will arrive deep inside your mind in a whole new world of comfort. The first point is the level of the mattress. You relax in the depth of your pillow and sink into the soft folds as you grow ten times relaxed.

The second level is the level of water. At this point, you can relax so deeply that you sink underneath the water surface. You should breathe easily. A big bubble of air follows you down and gives you what you need: the safest, fresh, and comfortable atmosphere to breathe. The water, like spring air, is moist, gentle, and sweet. You should slowly drift down like a leaf that is ten times more soothing than before.

The third level is the level of the siren. You will relax so deeply that you fall into a lovely jellyfish living in a palace on the seabed. As you merge with her beautiful body, you feel young and safe and relax ten times deeper.

The fourth point is the level of the seabed. You are going to sink deep into the warm sandy seabed coats. You're going to relax ten times more. Deeper and more profound. I the deepest sleep in your life, and yet you are still conscious. The world you discover here is fresh, infinite, the sky and the sea, peaceful and majestic, as the sun sets on the horizon.

Start to drift more profoundly into two levels any time you exhale. Inhale and go deeper and deeper as you exhale. Inhale allow your body to fill up with air and exhale more profound and more in-depth. Feel your hands and fingers get so heavy, hold to the material below, and get even more substantial. Imagine them sinking, heavy as two elephants bearing lead heads.

Experience this heaviness, this deep sense of calm flowing through your fingers and hands into your upper arms. Feel the active peace reaching out into your arms, back, ears, and head. Let this beautiful relaxed feeling spread through your eyebrows, your forehead, and your shoulders. Feel it trickle down your neck gradually. Allow your head and neck to sink into the pillow deeply. You relax more every time it falls in a little more. Feel the happiness going deeper and deeper, ten times deeper. You are now reaching the point of the mattress.

Through time you exhale, imagine that you are slipping into the world of harmony five times more profound. When your head was bubbled with beautiful fresh air, you float under the surface of the water. Peace is encircling you, spreading the strength of its warmth across your body. It floods into your subconscious as you exhale and sink into the water five times deeper. Too easy to think. Let your face and eyes shift the weight of this thoughtless love. It runs down your neck and extends into your chest from there. You get into your back and shoulders, elbows, knees, calves, ankles, feet, and toes. You come to the water level.

You have come more profound into the room of calm and peace around you and relax more and more as you sink into the warm and soothing water of relaxation. The pressure and the touch are right. You feel so comfortable; just relax more and more in your beautiful, welcoming environment. Steady and perfectly formed are your hands. You now approach the level of the siren.

Feel like you are turning into a sexy siren. You reached the stage of the siren. Feel how healthy, soothing, calming water is permeated by every pore of your lovely new body. Feels how the beauty of the cold, vast ocean suffuses every cell in your body. Respire the fresh, soothing air around you and feel like going down through the smooth water and into a sea of comfort more profound and more bottomless. The deeper you dive into the water, the better you feel.

Listen, when you exhale, to these numbers gurgling to your heart. With each amount, feel more profound and deeper, soothing and relaxed, reaching new levels of relaxation. 15-14-13-sink into the soothing ocean of rest more profound and deeper. 12-11—10—9—8—7—6—let it go all out—5—4—3,2—1 so dark, dreamy, and nebulous. Feel your sexy siren body sink to the ocean floor gently. The sandy bed is the smoothest and softest mattress you have ever had. Feel it with your hands and your feet. Lie down and touch your body with it. Start to sink deeper into the world's most cozy, soft bed. You have reached the condition of the seabed. You move further towards complete relaxation with every step. The level of calm and peace you can achieve is limitless. Breathe. Breathe. Relax. Relax.

Notice how the soothing water flows into your blood, hydrates your skin, and heals your internal organs, bones, and muscles. That cell in your body soaks up the world's best medicine and experiences an improvement in vital energy, vitality, and safety. Notice how the soothing water develops the characteristics and attitude and makes your hair, head, and body beautifully smooth. Feel a new serenity on your face to an enticing smile. Realize how much peace and confidence your body has relaxed. You can't be bothered by anything. You are powerful, lovely, and confident.

Prepare to return to the place and time you began your journey rejuvenated and refreshed. You're only going to be different. You return to your body after feeling the safe, revitalizing effects of your subconscious soothing ocean of relaxation. When you heard the last number, take another deep breath, and open your eyes. Open your eyes this time.

Once you return, you will drift into a lovely rejuvenating sleep or wake up to a new day. If you want to sleep first or wake up immediately, the new day will be met with positive energy, trust, and elegance. Ready? Ready? Let me now count you back to the surface as you plan for the flight. 10-10-9-8-7-6-5-3-2-1. Welcome back and thank for joining us on this journey to improve your life and make the world a better place.

CHAPTER SIX:
THE HEALING EFFECTS
OF SLEEP

Some believe the myth that we need less sleep as we age. We think sleeping three or four hours a night is enough to work correctly. If you wake up groggy or feel tired all day, you blame your busy lifestyle. They rely on caffeine to keep them alert and pledge to "catch up" during the weekend's sleep. The reality is that children, adolescents, and adults need more than a few hours of sleep each night. Chronic diseases, such as depression, hypertension, diabetes, and obesity, are more likely to occur in people who lack sleep. Indeed, rest is increasingly seen as critical to public health due to insufficient sleep concerning motor vehicle crashes, industrial incidents, and medical and other occupational mistakes.

The Importance of Sleep

Like food and exercise, sleep is essential to optimal health and happiness. While you rest, your brain stays active and is responsible for a wide range of biological maintenance tasks, which keeps your mind and body functioning and prepares you for the day ahead. The body needs time to heal, refresh, and detox properly. It is not enough time for your body to sleep just a few hours to get your body ready to work at its best. Some of the risks involved with inadequate sleep are as follows:

Short-term memory loss

Sleep privation will affect the memory for a short time and hurt your thought. You can forget about a task or stop halfway, forgetting what the original job was.

Depression

You may not be able to complete simple tasks if you lack motivation. The lack of energy and the loss of focus will contribute to a negative picture of yourself.

Weak Immune System

The sleep of the body is when tissues heal and rebuild, bone and muscle development, and the immune system is improved.

Metabolism and weight

Deprivation of chronic sleep can cause weight gain by disrupting the processing and storage of carbohydrates and altering hormone levels that influence our appetite.

Mood

Sleep loss can lead to irritability, impatience, lack of concentration, and mood. Too little sleep can also make you too exhausted to do stuff.

Cardiovascular Health

Hypertension elevated stress hormone levels, and irregular heartbeats have been associated with severe sleep disorders.

How much sleep is enough?

According to the National Sleep Foundation, although the needs for sleep differ a little from person to person, most healthy adults require between 7 and 9 hours of sleep per night to perform their best. The Foundation recommends that children in schools (5-10 years) require 10-11 hours of sleep every day, and teenagers (10-17 years) need 8.5-9.5 hours.

According to the National Health Interview results, almost 30% of adults reported an average of six hours or less per day of sleep. Just 31% of high school students reported sleeping for an average school night for at least 8 hours.

One of the biggest myths is that people can "take" sleep by sleeping during the weekend. It turns outweighs not that easy to recover from a chronic lack of sleep. It is not enough to get two good nights of sleep to pay off long-term debt. While extra sleep can be given a temporary boost, the day wears down your efficiency and strength.

How to get enough sleep hygiene

Tips For the sake of good sleeping habits and daily sleep,

"Sleep hygiene" is known. With this little effort and practice, the following tips on sleep hygiene will help you sleep well:

- Go to bed every night simultaneously and get yourself up every morning. Coherence is critical. When you have a regular sleep schedule, you're much more rested and energized than sleeping at different times for the same number of hours.
- Regular physical activity can contribute to sleep promotion, but a few hours before going to bed will be prevented.
- Avoid big meals before going to bed.
- Avoid close bedtime, caffeine, and alcohol.
- Evite nicotine.
- Don't watch TV, cook, work, or use your room computers. Clear from the bedroom, all televisions, laptops, and other "gadgets."

- Make sure the room is calm, dark, and soothing, not too hot or too cold.

- If you're incredibly tired and can't function during the day, a short nap can help to relax and reset. Reduce your rest to thirty minutes as longer sleep can interfere with your sleep at night.

Try integrating the treatment of your mind and therapies like yoga, meditation, acupuncture, reiki, reflexology, and massage into your daily routine as well as having good sleep habits. Research has shown that these treatments relax the mind and ready the body for restorative sleep.

Relax with meditation and guided imagery

One thing that keeps people alert at night is that their mind is concerned. The brain releases the natural tranquilizing chemicals by using visualization for relaxation, and meditation, which renders directed imaging a usual way of reducing stress-related conditions, such as headaches, high blood pressure, pre-menstrual stress, and other stress-related psychological conditions.

Yoga

Research suggests that this ancient exercise can help fight against insomnia, reduce tension, and avoid aches and pains that can leave you tossing and turning all night long.

Reiki / Touch Healing Therapy

Reiki has based on Western philosophy that energy helps your natural healing ability. Reiki is a healing touch therapy. Reiki is a healing activity in which practitioners lightly or just above the individual to promote their healing response. Reiki sessions will help you relax and relax to prepare the way to better sleep.

Acupuncture

Acupuncture has a nervous system relaxing effect. It enhances sleep patterns by the clearing of muscle and nerve channel obstructions, encourages the release of oxygen-enriched energy, and relaxes the body.

Reflexology

operated by stress relaxation and suppressed energy release. The reflex point in the middle of the top pad in each broad toe refers to the pineal gland. A tiny cone-like organ that releases the hormone melatonin is the pineal gland. Since melatonin affects the sleep pattern of an individual, healthy sleep must maintain a balanced level.

Sleep - Why It Should Top Your Priority List

Most believe that rest is a waste of time. Nothing is going on, after all. All those hours in the night when you could do stuff! Here's why it's not only wrong; it's a risky line of thought.

It's not that nothing is going on during the night. A lot is going on! It's not that you go from the priority list of your body during exercise to no priority list during sleep. Alternatively, rest implies a change from the behaviors that reign during your day to the activities that rule during the night.

During sleep, the body allows all behaviors that do not occur in active mode "rest-and-digest" or "beat and raise." All those resources that were moved into operation are now allocated to these other roles during restful sleep. Are there any examples? The body builds bone in the night, rebuilding tissue, washing waste, combating bacteria, eliminating toxins, creating new cells.

When this turn isn't made in your automatic nervous system, you will eventually weaken and then burn out your pituitary gland, thyroid, adrenal glands, and gonads. This is achieved through two aspects of your automatic system that activate and inhibit those endocrine glands. It galvanizes the muscle system and the ability to react physically in the daytime or active mode. Their focus prioritizes cleaning and maintenance during the night or sleep mode.

Don't give this second agenda enough time, and you and your body are exhausted by the fact that different functions start to fail. As you start, do, do, fix, and repair your physical condition gets worse. This is the way it ends up in an early grave with a harrowing ride on the road.

The body requires much more extended periods of restorative-healing mode in cases, including childbirth, where the agency has a long list of recovery-repair work to do, including rehabilitation from emotional or physical shock or trauma.

During sleep, they are tasks that do not require quick responses, such as those controlled by your active-day (or sympathetic nervous system) agenda.

The rest healing (or parasympathetic mode) stimulates five body systems:

- Lungs
- Liver
- Intestinal tract
- Pancreas
- Bronchial muscles

While, it inhibits these five glands:

- The adrenal
- Hypophysis
- The nucleus

- The thyroid
- The ovaries

Why can't you sleep?

The common causes of the disease are:

- Food allergies
- Heavy metals
- Petroleum solvencies

-Bacteria

-Viruses

-Yeasts

-Lyme vectors and cofactors

-Parasites

-Mold

- Physical toxicity
- EMF exposure (wireless internet links, mobile phones, smart meters, microwave stoves, etc.)

- Medicines that activate your sympathetic system or inhibit your sympathetic system (the terms of online search indicate which ones).

Promoting restful sleep

Many necessary measures are available to support good night's sleep:

- Avoid the main food intolerances; they are the lead producers of sympathetic superiority that is the different autonomic nervous mode to be used to cure sleep.

- Do not eat stimulants in the middle of the afternoon. You can instead drink herbal teas soothing (chamomile or lemon bake are two examples of nerve soothing) or peppermint to improve your digestion.

- Through your consumption of alkaline mineral products, as they help to slow down things, particularly if your body feels like racing.

- Several sources are potassium, iodine, kelp, calcium, magnesium, and vitamin D. African berries, orange juice, bananas, dates, raisins, potatoes, and yams are a rich source of food.

- Prevent overuse of sugar-for many reasons, this is always a good idea, but sugar is the primary cause of potassium depletion in terms of sleep.

- Consider using diuretics and blood pressure drugs, as they also deplete potassium wherever possible.

CONCLUSION

Yoga Nidra is the most profound type of relaxation-experienced during meditation by Yogis. It is described as bringing profound calmness and clarity to mind and is often referred to as' yogic sleep.' In the state of Yoga Nidra, you are over waking, dreaming, and sleeping as you are awake.

Yoga Nidra can be hard to achieve, but it can occur in every meditation session, with regular practice and a dedicated mindset, if a practitioner so chooses. Once you practice Yoga Nidra steadily, it gives the practitioner a profound peace and calm that transcends into everyday life. Also, strenuous psychological and physical tasks do not feel as exhausting when you are relaxed.